101 slide tests for the MRCP

101
slide tests
for the MRCP

Jonathan L Brown MA MRCP
Registrar in Medicine
The London Hospital Medical Rotation
London UK

David M Hansell MB MRCP
Registrar in Radiology
Westminster Hospital
London UK

Churchill Livingstone
EDINBURGH LONDON MELBOURNE AND NEW YORK 1986

CHURCHILL LIVINGSTONE
Medical Division of Longman Group Limited

Distributed in the United States of America by
Churchill Livingstone Inc., 1560 Broadway, New York,
N.Y. 10036, and by associated companies, branches
and representatives throughout the world.

First published 1986

ISBN 0 443 03465 6

British Library Cataloguing in Publication Data

Brown, Jonathan L.
   101 slides for the MRCP.
   1. Pathology—Pictorial works
   I. Title   II. Hansell, David M.
   616'.0022'2   RB33

Library of Congress Cataloging in Publication Data

Brown, Jonathan L.
   101 slides for the MRCP.
   1. Internal medicine—Examinations, questions, etc.
   2. Internal medicine—Atlases.   3. Pathology—Slides
(Photography)   I. Hansell, David M.   II. Title.
III. Title: One hundred one slides for the MRCP.
IV. Title: One hundred and one slides for the MRCP.
[DNLM: 1. Medicine—atlases.   2. Medicine—examination
questions.   W 18 D878z]
RC58.B76   1986   616'.0076   85-19556

Produced by Longman Group (FE) Limited
Printed in Hong Kong

Preface

This book is aimed at postgraduates who are preparing for Part Two of the Membership Diploma of the Royal College of Physicians and similar examinations now being held overseas. In the 'projected material' section of the Membership examination, a slide is shown for a two-minute period, during which candidates give written answers to short questions in a booklet. Twenty slides in all are projected and a signal is given half a minute before each slide is changed. Common clinical conditions make up the majority of slides shown although some unexpectedly esoteric material has been used in the past.

Candidates can never hope to be completely prepared for this section, since the Royal Colleges have access to a vast collection of material which is ever-changing. In addition, there is no doubt that this is a somewhat artificial way of looking at clinical material and radiographs; hence familiarity with as many examples as possible, in the form of slides or photographs, will make this section less daunting. For this reason we make no apology for adding another book to the selection already available.

The ratio of clinical pictures to radiographs and other material (including histopathological sections and blood films) in this book is approximately the same as in the examination itself. The clinical information given with each slide in the examination is kept to essentials, a style which we have adopted in this book. Any idea that the correct answer can be deduced from the picture caption alone is false. There may be more than one correct answer to some questions and we have given all the options without necessarily listing them in order of preference. In some questions we have asked for short lists of causes of the conditions shown. However, most questions in the examination require only a single answer. The discussions which follow each answer should not be regarded as comprehensive and we have put more emphasis on those conditions which may be less familiar.

In this compilation, an important consideration has been to keep costs to a minimum, bearing in mind that it will have limited usefulness to those fortunate candidates who will use it no more than once. The quality of reproduction on the printed page can never achieve that of the original slides and radiographs, but candidates can be assured that all material used in the examination is meticulously chosen and presented.

London   D.M.H.
1986   J.L.B.

Acknowledgements

This book contains slides and radiographs from many colleagues' collections and we are grateful for their permission to use them. The Haematology Department of University College Hospital has kindly lent us a number of blood films. Acknowledgement is also due to the authors of hundreds of review articles: we have drawn freely upon their collective wisdom.

We would particularly like to thank Dr Margaret Phelan, Dr David Rampton, and P.H. for their advice in the preparation of the text. Mr Keith Duguid and the Department of Medical Photography of Westminster Medical School have generously given us their time and expertise in the production of the illustrations. We are indebted to Miss M.A. Moule for the long hours she spent typing a mercurial manuscript. The completion of this book was helped considerably by the encouragement of the publishing staff at Churchill Livingstone.

Question 1

1. What are the two abnormalities in this picture?
2. What is the diagnosis?

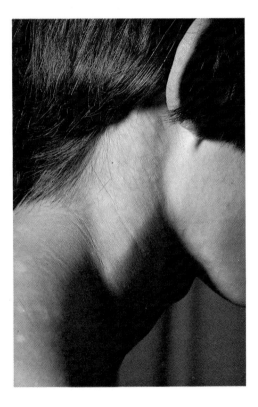

Answer to question 1

1. (a) Hypertrophy of the great auricular nerve.
   (b) Hypopigmented patches over the shoulder.
2. Tuberculoid leprosy.

The clinical course of leprosy is dependent on host immunity. Patients with a high level of immunity (lepromin-positive) develop the tuberculoid form of the disease with hypopigmented anaesthetic skin patches and enlargement of peripheral nerves. The histological features are of epithelioid and giant cell granulomas with relatively few bacilli.

Those with poorer immunity develop the lepromatous form with symmetrical macules, papules and nodules. The lesions are teeming with bacilli and tend not to be anaesthetic. The lepromin test is negative and nerve thickening is a late feature.

Between these polar forms lie borderline conditions, which, in the absence of treatment, tend to downgrade to the lepromatous form.

Question 2

This patient has multiple sebaceous cysts and lipomas on his skin.
1. What is the diagnosis?
2. What is the main complication?

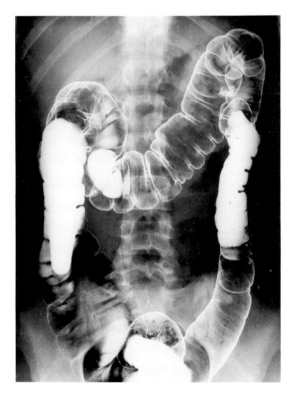

Answer to question 2

1. Gardner's syndrome.
2. Malignant change of colonic polyps.

Gardner's syndrome comprises adenomatous polyposis of the colon and soft tissue tumours (lipomas, sebaceous cysts and fibromas) with or without osteomas of the skull and long bones. Rarer associations of Gardner's syndrome include (a) thyroid carcinoma (b) duodenal adenomas capable of malignant change (c) periampullary carcinoma in the pancreas.

The distinction between familial polyposis coli and Gardner's syndrome has been questioned, since close examination of patients with so-called 'familial polyposis coli' often reveals soft tissue tumours.

The malignant potential of the colonic polyps in both conditions is identical and the treatment of total colectomy is mandatory. Follow-up sigmoidoscopy every 6 months is essential if the rectum has been left for an ileorectal anastomosis.

Question 3

1. What is the abnormality?
2. What is the likely cause?

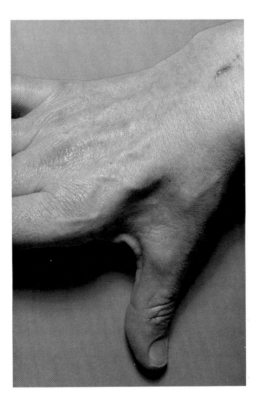

Answer to question 3

1. Wasting of 1st dorsal interosseous muscle.
2. Ulnar nerve lesion.

The small muscles of the hand take their root value from T1. They are supplied by the ulnar nerve, with the exception of abductor pollicis brevis, flexor pollicis brevis, opponens pollicis and the lateral two lumbricals. Abductor pollicis brevis is almost invariably innervated by the median nerve.

Ulnar nerve lesions commonly occur with a fracture of the medial epicondyle at the elbow or from the continuous minor trauma associated with cubitus valgus. The ulnar tunnel syndrome may arise from a compression band at this site. The nerve may also be damaged by injury to the wrist. Paradoxically, the deformity is greater in low lesions which leave the ulnar half of flexor digitorum profundus unopposed by the lumbricals and interossei. The ring and little fingers are hyperextended at the metacarpophalangeal joints and flexed at the interphalangeal joints.

A true claw hand occurs with a root or cord lesion, or combined median and ulnar nerve disorders. Recognised causes include motor neurone disease, dystrophia myotonica, ascending polyneuritis, polio and leprosy. Klumpke's paralysis, thoracic outlet obstruction (Pancoast's tumour, cervical rib) and syringomyelia make up the proximal causes. Volkmann's ischaemic contracture may lead to an identical appearance.

The small muscles of the hand are frequently wasted in rheumatoid arthritis. This may be due to a combination of disuse, peripheral neuropathy, nerve entrapment and myopathy.

Question 4

This is the chest radiograph of a 14-year-old boy.
1. What is the diagnosis?
2. Name five complications of this disorder.

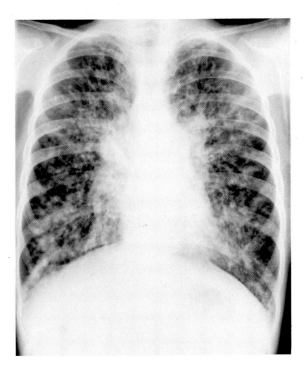

Answer to question 4

1. Cystic fibrosis.
2. (a) Meconium ileus. (b) Infertility in males.
   (c) Bronchiectasis. (d) Emphysema. (e) Pneumothorax.
   (f) Nasal polyps. (g) Abnormal glucose tolerance test.
   (h) Steatorrhoea. (i) Arthralgia. (j) Skin rashes.
   (k) Hypertrophic osteoarthropathy. (l) Progressive
   cirrhosis. (m) Heat stroke.

The earliest radiographic finding in cystic fibrosis is bronchial wall thickening seen predominantly in the upper zones. Other features are ring shadows due to bronchiectatic airways and generalised mottling caused by small areas of consolidation around small bronchi. Hyperinflation of the lungs is an almost invariable finding due to extensive obstruction of medium and small airways. As the disease progresses bilateral hilar prominence may occur due to either lymph node enlargement resulting from chronic pulmonary infection or pulmonary artery dilatation secondary to pulmonary hypertension.

The clinical manifestations and complications of cystic fibrosis are legion. Infertility is extremely common in male patients (over 95%). Pneumothoraces are not uncommon in older patients and if there is any clinical suspicion an expiratory chest radiograph should be requested.

Question 5

1. What is the cause of this marrow appearance?
2. Name four biochemical abnormalities associated with this condition.

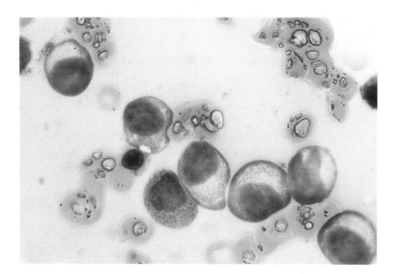

Answer to question 5

1. Myeloma.
2. (a) Elevated blood globulin.
   (b) M-band on protein electrophoresis.
   (c) Bence-Jones proteinuria.
   (d) Immune paresis (reduction in immunoglobulin
       subclasses other than the paraprotein).
   (e) Hyponatraemia.
   (f) Hypercalcaemia.
   (g) Hyperuricaemia.
   (h) Uraemia.

Myelomatosis results from a monoclonal proliferation of plasma cells. The associated immune paresis distinguishes this malignant condition from benign gammopathy, a common finding in the elderly.

Typical presentations include bone pain (particularly lumbosacral), pathological fractures, haemorrhage, anaemia and recurrent infection. Rarely the presentation is with symptoms of hypercalcaemia or uraemia. Renal failure can occur as a result of direct tubular damage from light chains, hypercalcaemia, hyperuricaemia or amyloid.

The diagnosis is confirmed by examination of the bone marrow, which shows a diffuse proliferation of plasma cells. These have basophilic cytoplasm, and an eccentric nucleus, often with a perinuclear halo. Light chain proteinuria (Bence-Jones) is present in 70% of cases. This protein gives a positive reaction with salicylsulphonic acid and coagulates at 45–60°C when the urine is warmed. The protein dissolves on boiling but precipitates again when cooled. λ-Chain proteinuria has a worse prognosis than κ-chain proteinuria.

The disease is invariably fatal. A combination of melphalan, cyclophosphamide, corticosteroids and radiotherapy is used for palliation. Renal damage can be minimised by reducing tumour mass with chemotherapy, removing light chains with plasma exchange and maintaining a high fluid intake. Allopurinol is given for the treatment of hyperuricaemia.

Question 6

This is the wrist of an epileptic child.
What is the likely cause of this appearance?

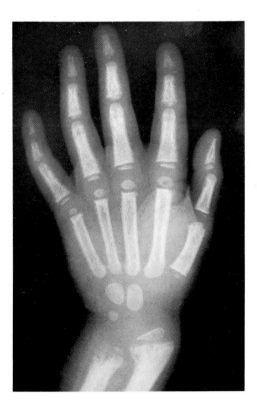

Answer to question 6

Anticonvulsant rickets.

The appearance of this unfused wrist is typical of rickets. There is irregular mineralisation and widening of the metaphysis, which is cupped and ragged. The area of provisional calcification is absent, resulting in displacement of the epiphysis from the shaft of the bone.

The prolonged use of anticonvulsants has been shown to cause osteomalacia, of varying severity, in 65% of institutionalised epileptics. Before incriminating anticonvulsants as the cause of rickets, other causes such as dietary deficiency of vitamin D, malabsorption and renal disease should be excluded.

Rickets or osteomalacia caused by anticonvulsant therapy is partially due to the induction of hepatic enzymes which degrade vitamin D_3 and 25-hydroxycholecalciferol to inactive metabolites. In addition, phenytoin has been shown to reduce intestinal calcium absorption. Interestingly, osteomalacia has been reported following the long-term administration of rifampicin; again, hepatic enzyme induction is thought to be responsible.

Question 7

This patient, without a refractive error, has noticed a
deterioration in visual acuity.
1. Name two abnormalities on the fundus.
2. What treatment is required?

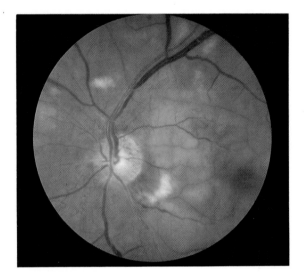

Answer to question 7

1. (a) Soft exudates (retinal infarcts).
   (b) New vessel formation.
2. Urgent ophthalmic referral for laser photocoagulation.

The picture is typical of proliferative diabetic retinopathy. The new vessels growing from the disc are particularly liable to cause haemorrhage, leading to retinal detachment with collapse of the vitreous body. The 'cotton-wool' spots represent infarcts of the nerve layer and with venous beading and reduplication are the hallmark of the pre-proliferative phase.

Oedematous maculopathy may be difficult to detect with the ophthalmoscope, but its presence is suggested by a loss in visual acuity unaffected by the pinhole test. Focal maculopathy is associated with hard exudates in a circular distribution around the macula, and an ischaemic maculopathy with the co-existence of 'cotton-wool' spots.

Background retinopathy is characterised by microaneurysms and haemorrhages (dot and blot appearance), with hard exudates (accumulations of lipid) around leaky vessels.

Vascular abnormalities are more readily identified with fluorescein angiography and this technique facilitates treatment. Proliferative retinopathy requires panretinal photocoagulation, which is usually spread over several sessions. Several thousand laser burns are focussed on the peripheral retina, avoiding the macula and disc. Focal maculopathy may be treated by ablating the middle of circinate exudates, and oedematous maculopathy by arranging a grid of burns over the macula, avoiding the fovea.

Hypertension, cigarette smoking, excessive alcohol intake and poor glycaemic control are established risk factors for diabetic retinopathy.

Question 8

This is the CT scan of a 14-year-old patient who presented with symptoms of raised intracranial pressure and a bitemporal lower quadrantic visual field defect.
What is the likely diagnosis?

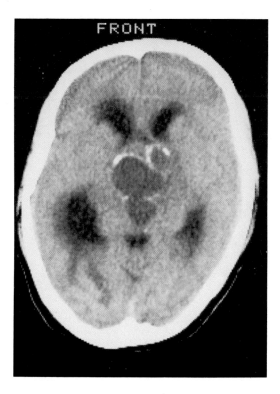

Answer to question 8

Craniopharyngioma.

The unenhanced CT scan shows a mid-line cystic lesion containing calcium. It is suprasellar and from the history is compressing the optic chiasma from above. At this age a craniopharyngioma is by far the most likely diagnosis. Calcification is seen in over 75% of cases. A skull radiograph may, in addition, show an enlarged pituitary fossa if there is intrasellar extension or flattening of the dorsum sellae. There is ventricular dilatation in this scan due to obstruction of the third ventricle by upward extension of the craniopharyngioma.

Craniopharyngiomas are squamous cell tumours which arise from the remnants of Rathke's pouch. Because of their position the clinical presentations are protean and to some extent depend on the patient's age.

Children
Pituitary dwarfism.
Symptoms of raised intracranial pressure.
Visual field defects.
Papilloedema or optic atrophy.
Hypothalamic syndromes (e.g. obesity, somnolence).

Adults
Variable pituitary dysfunction.
Progressive visual failure.
Slight spastic weakness of the legs.
Disturbances of temperature regulation (hypothalamic involvement).

Elderly
Dementia due to hydrocephalus.
Progressive visual failure.

Total surgical removal is followed by recurrence in up to 10% of cases. The tumour is relatively insensitive to radiotherapy.

Question 9

1. What complication of alcoholism has occurred?
2. How is the diagnosis confirmed?
3. What treatment is required?

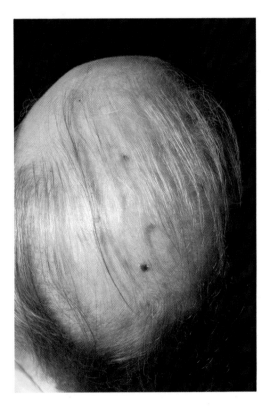

Answer to question 9

1. Porphyria cutanea tarda.
2. Detection of urinary uroporphyrin.
3. Complete withdrawal of alcohol and regular venesection.

This condition is an acquired porphyria resulting from chemical liver damage, the commonest toxin being alcohol. The liver invariably shows a siderosis and in most cases the serum iron is elevated. Both alcohol and iron can induce amino-laevulinic acid synthetase, the first enzyme in the biosynthetic pathway of haem synthesis from glycine and succinyl-CoA. Reduced activity of enzymes lower in the pathway result in an accumulation of uro- and coproporphyrins which may be detected in the urine.

Acute neurological attacks are not a feature of porphyria cutanea tarda. Patients with this condition present with haemorrhagic and crusted lesions on light-exposed areas which heal to leave a shallow scar.

Remission may occur with complete abstinence from alcohol, and lowering of serum iron with regular venesection.

Question 10

This is a lymph node biopsy from a patient who has painful eyes and a facial nerve palsy.
1. What does the biopsy show?
2. What syndrome does this patient have?

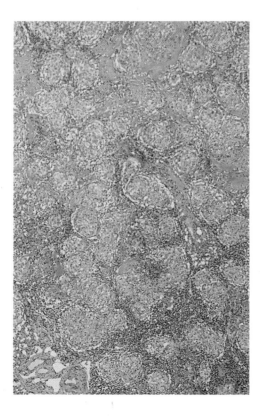

Answer to question 10

1. Sarcoid granulomas.
2. Heerfordt's syndrome.

There are numerous granulomas replacing the normal lymph node architecture. The lesions consist of epithelioid cells (histiocytes) with a few giant cells and some peripheral lymphocytes. These granulomas are all of approximately the same size and do not show central caseation: these features suggest sarcoidosis rather than tuberculosis. The distinction from tuberculous granulomas can be difficult if there is minimal central necrosis. However, in sarcoidosis the reticulin framework is preserved in the central necrosis whereas in the caseation of tuberculosis this is lost.

Heerfordt's syndrome (uveoparotid fever) is the triad of parotid enlargement, anterior uveitis, and facial nerve palsy; this may be the first manifestation of sarcoidosis.

Question 11

1. What is the cause of this appearance?
2. How is it treated?

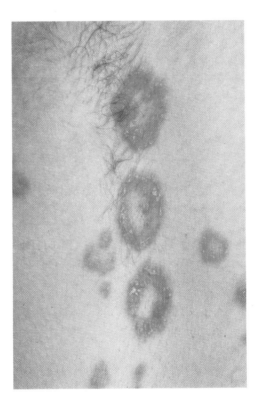

Answer to question 11

1. Tinea corporis (ringworm).
2. Griseofulvin.

The lesions of tinea corporis usually originate in the axillae or groins; typically they have a pruritic, elevated and advancing edge with central clearing. These lesions may be confused with psoriasis or seborrhoeic dermatitis, but the diagnosis is revealed by an examination of scrapings taken from the advancing edge.

Griseofulvin is the treatment of choice for widespread ringworm and should be taken for 6 weeks. Absorption is increased if the drug is administered with a fatty meal.

Question 12

This patient presented with peripheral oedema, weight loss and lassitude. She was found to have hypoalbuminaemia.
1. What is the diagnosis?
2. Name four possible causes.

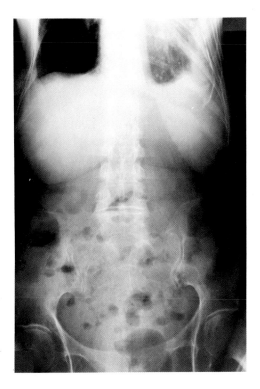

Answer to question 12

1. Constrictive pericarditis.
2. (a) Post-infective, e.g. Coxsackie B, tuberculosis, infectious mononucleosis, staphylococcus.
   (b) Traumatic haemopericarditis.
   (c) Post-irradiation.
   (d) Connective tissue diseases.
   (e) Infiltrating carcinoma (rarely calcified).

Pericardial calcification is diagnostic but it is found in less than one-half of all cases of constrictive pericarditis. Other features which might be seen on an abdominal radiograph are hepatomegaly and ascites. The diagnosis of cirrhosis may be mistakenly made if the cardiac signs are unconvincing and pericardial calcification is absent.

Constrictive pericarditis is not always preceded by an obvious precipitating factor. The symptoms of malaise and anorexia often predominate and patients may be severely debilitated. Ascites is usually more pronounced than peripheral oedema. Breathlessness and orthopnoea both occur in the later stages. However, episodes of left ventricular failure are not a feature of constrictive pericarditis.

A protein-losing enteropathy due to impaired lymphatic drainage of the small intestine may result in hypoalbuminaemia. Frank nephrotic syndrome may develop in more severe cases of constrictive pericarditis.

Mild constrictive pericarditis is not necessarily progressive and asymptomatic patients do not require treatment. Diuretics and sodium restriction may control symptoms, but pericardiectomy is the definitive treatment for patients with severe constriction.

Question 13

1. Name this lesion.
2. What is the cause?
3. Name three other abnormalities that may be visible on inspection of this patient.

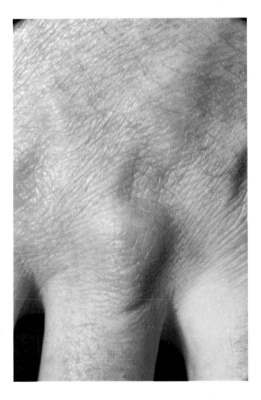

Answer to question 13

1. Tendon xanthoma.
2. Familial hypercholesterolaemia.
3. (a) Tuberous xanthomata.
   (b) Xanthelasma palpebrarum.
   (c) Corneal arcus.

Familial hypercholesterolaemia is inherited as an autosomal dominant condition and affects 1 in 500 people. Diminished activity of peripheral low density lipoprotein receptors is responsible. Untreated homozygotes rarely survive the third decade and half the heterozygous males have manifestations of ischaemic heart disease by the age of fifty.

Tendon xanthomata are found within the Achilles tendon and the extensor tendons of the hand over the metacarpal heads.

Those affected should be advised against smoking and be prescribed a low cholesterol diet. Oral contraceptives should not be given to women. Administration of the bile acid sequestrant cholestyramine has been shown to reduce serum cholesterol and cardiac mortality.

More aggressive management is appropriate for the homozygous patient and this may include ileal bypass surgery and plasma exchange.

Question 14

What is the likely cause of this radiological appearance?

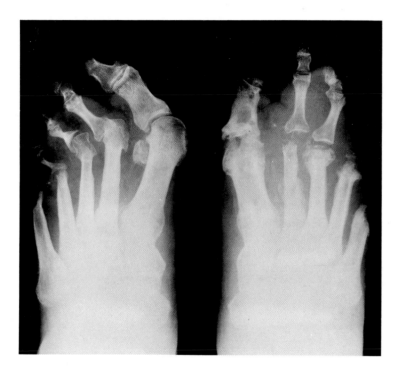

Answer to question 14

Diabetes mellitus.

The diabetic foot has a characteristic radiological appearance. Resorption of the metatarsal heads and disorganisation of the metatarsophalangeal joints with or without the changes of osteomyelitis are the usual appearances of the anaesthetic diabetic foot. In addition, arterial calcification may be seen; gas in the soft tissues is a sinister sign and signifies gangrene. In more advanced cases severe disability results from the neuropathic (Charcot) disorganisation of the intertarsal and ankle joints.

The changes are due to peripheral neuropathy and vascular insufficiency possibly due to shunting. Gangrenous toes in the presence of normal pedal pulses are not uncommon and reflect predominantly microvascular disease.

Question 15

This is the bone marrow of a patient who presented with a
haemoglobin of 6.2 g/dl and shortness of breath.
1. What treatment is required?
2. Name three other tests that will help with the further
   management of this patient.

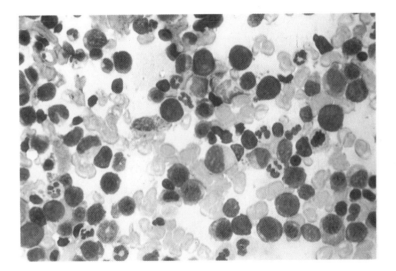

Answer to question 15

1. Parenteral hydroxocobalamin and oral folic acid.
2. (a) Serum B_{12} assay.
   (b) Red cell folate assay.
   (c) Auto-antibody screen (intrinsic factor, gastric parietal cell).
   (d) Schilling test.

The marrow is frankly megaloblastic. The erythroid cells are larger than their normoblastic counterparts and the nuclei have a stippled appearance. There is a disproportionate increase in primitive forms. The myeloid series show a delay in nuclear maturation.

A typical peripheral blood film in this condition reveals a macrocytic anaemia, anisocytosis, poikilocytosis, nucleated red cells, leucopenia, thrombocytopenia and hypersegmented neutrophils. Serum bilirubin, lactate dehydrogenase and urinary urobilin are elevated.

Treatment should be initiated with hydroxocobalamin and folic acid as soon as a megaloblastic marrow is diagnosed. The results of vitamin B_{12} and folate estimations are usually delayed. A low red cell folate level is required to confirm significant depletion, as a low serum folate level only indicates negative folate balance.

Intrinsic factor and gastric parietal cell antibodies are detectable in most cases of Addisonian pernicious anaemia. The Schilling test helps to confirm this diagnosis and to distinguish between this condition and other megaloblastic anaemias caused by intestinal abnormalities.

Question 16

This 45-year-old patient presented with recurrent epistaxis and renal failure.
1. What is the most likely diagnosis?
2. What is the treatment for this condition?

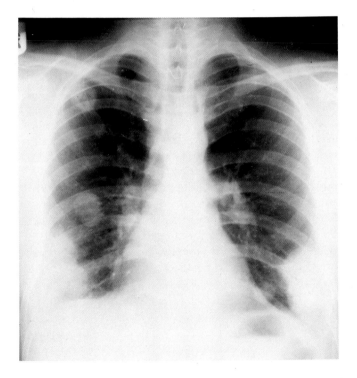

Answer to question 16

1. Wegener's granulomatosis.
2. Immunosuppressive therapy including cyclophosphamide.

Wegener's granulomatosis is a multisystem disease in which the respiratory tract and kidneys are affected by granulomatous inflammation and a necrotising vasculitis. The disease usually occurs in males over 40 years old.

The earliest features of the disease involve the upper respiratory tract (e.g. sinusitis, epistaxis and otitis media). This is followed by symptoms of fever, arthralgia, pleuritic chest pain and haemoptysis. Renal involvement occurs at a late stage and is present in 90% of patients. Less common features are (a) iritis (b) pericarditis (c) coronary arteritis (d) mononeuritis multiplex (e) skin petechiae and ulceration.

There are no specific laboratory tests for Wegener's granulomatosis, but the clinical features in conjunction with the histological picture of both vasculitis and granulomatous inflammation usually allow a definitive diagnosis to be made.

The prognosis without treatment is very poor. With cytotoxic treatment more than 90% will go into remission and a substantial number will not relapse.

Question 17

1. What is this condition?
2. With what disease is it associated?
3. Name three other clinical features of this disease.

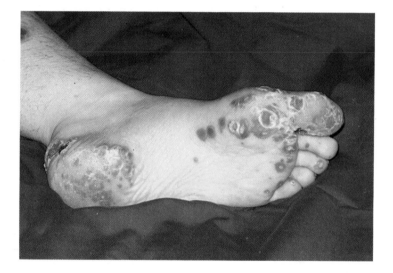

Answer to question 17

1. Keratoderma blenorrhagica.
2. Reiter's disease.
3. (a) Skeletal: polyarthritis, sacroileitis, tendonitis and fasciitis.
   (b) Ocular: conjunctivitis, episcleritis, uveitis.
   (c) Urethritis (even in cases precipitated by dysentery).
   (d) Mucous membranes: circinate balanitis, buccal ulceration.
   (e) Others: carditis, pleurisy and neurological disturbances (all rare).

The clinical triad of urethritis, conjunctivitis and polyarthritis make up Reiter's disease, a condition almost exclusive to males. There is a strong association with the inheritance of HLA-B27. The disease is usually preceded by a non-specific genital infection (particularly chlamydial), but may follow bacterial dysentery, the commonest causes being *Shigella, Salmonella* or *Yersinia.*

The knee is the most consistently affected joint and synovial fluid aspirate is sterile with a high leucocyte count. Achilles tendonitis and plantar fasciitis contribute significantly to the patient's immobility.

In most cases the condition resolves spontaneously, but the appearance of keratoderma blenorrhagica (macules and scaly pustules resembling pustular psoriasis) predicts a chronic relapsing course and ultimately joint destruction.

Question 18

This patient has noticed grittiness of the eyes and weight-loss despite a good appetite.
What is the likely diagnosis?

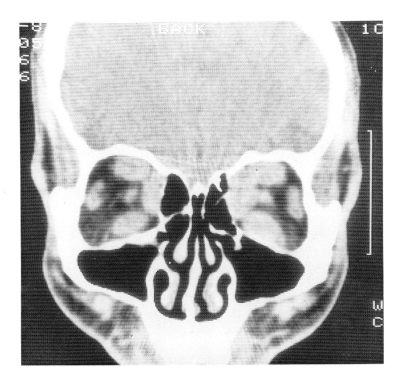

Answer to question 18

Thyroid eye disease.

The CT scan demonstrates swelling of all the extraocular muscles, which is characteristic of established thyroid eye disease. The extraocular myositis is now thought to be mediated by a specific ophthalmopathic autoantibody directed at a retro-orbital muscle antigen. This antibody may or may not co-exist with thyroid autoantibodies. Thus the typical eye changes of Graves' thyrotoxicosis may occur in the absence of clinical or biochemical thyrotoxicosis; this is referred to as 'endocrine exophthalmos' and follow-up of these patients is necessary as a few become either thyrotoxic or hypothyroid.

The spectrum of eye involvement in thyrotoxicosis has been usefully graded in the Werner classification:

0 No eye signs or symptoms.
1 Eye signs only (e.g. lid retraction or proptosis up to 22 mm). No symptoms.
2 Soft tissue involvement (e.g. symptomatic eyelid oedema).
3 Proptosis greater than 22 mm.
4 Extraocular muscle involvement.
5 Corneal injury.
6 Optic nerve damage and blindness.

Question 19

1. What is this condition?
2. Name five causes.

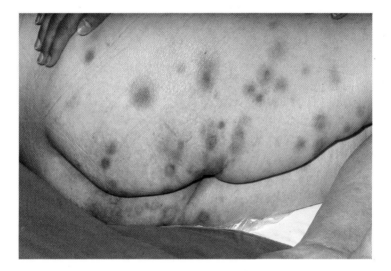

Answer to question 19

1. Erythema multiforme.
2. (a) Infections: herpes simplex, mycoplasma pneumoniae, streptococci.
   (b) Drugs: sulphonamides, penicillin, barbiturates, phenytoin, aspirin.
   (c) Malignancy.

The lesions have a symmetrical distribution and are found around the mucous membranes and extensor surfaces of the limbs. They have a target appearance and the centre may contain a bulla. In its most severe form the condition is known as the 'Stevens-Johnson syndrome'.
   In 50% of cases the cause is unknown; an association has been described with internal malignancy and is occasionally precipitated by radiotherapy.

Question 20

This man presented with a haematemesis.
What is the likely diagnosis?

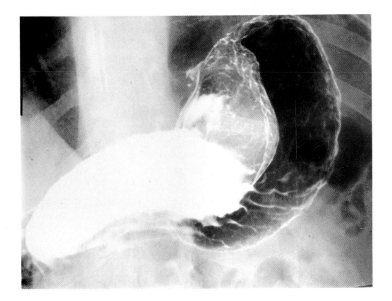

Answer to question 20

Leiomyoma.

The most likely cause of the enormous filling defect in the stomach is a leiomyoma. Clinically the patient may present with a brisk gastrointestinal haemorrhage or a palpable epigastric mass. Less likely causes are other benign tumours such as an adenoma, lipoma, or Schwannoma.

The leiomyoma arises from the muscle layer of the stomach and the overlying mucosa is stretched causing central ulceration which is said to be characteristic. 10% undergo sarcomatous change; the likelihood of this occurring increases with the size of the leiomyoma.

Question 21

1. What is the abnormality?
2. Name four causes.

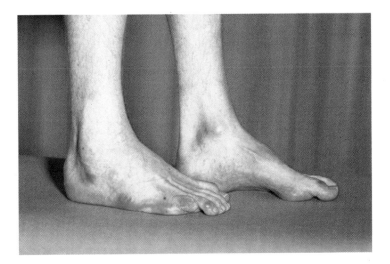

Answer to question 21

1. Pes cavus.
2. (a) Spina bifida.
   (b) Myelodysplasia.
   (c) Poliomyelitis.
   (d) Friedreich's ataxia.
   (e) Peroneal muscular atrophy.
   (f) Syringomyelia.
   (g) Homocystinuria.

Pes cavus (claw foot) occurs in conditions that affect the balance of the intrinsic foot muscles. The longitudinal arch becomes exaggerated, with hyperextension of the toes at the metatarsophalangeal joints and flexion at the proximal and distal interphalangeal joints. Some familial cases associated with a short plantar fascia occur in the absence of neurological disease.

Question 22

1. What condition is associated with this appearance?
2. Name three tests that will confirm the diagnosis.

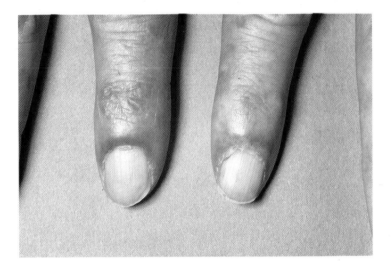

Answer to question 22

1. Dermatomyositis.
2. (a) Biochemical: elevated transaminases and creatine phosphokinase.
   (b) Histological:
      (i) Muscle biopsy – signs of degeneration, regeneration, necrosis and fibrosis, with a mononuclear cell infiltrate.
      (ii) Skin biopsy – oedema and focal arteriolar fibrinoid degeneration (this may be distinguished from systemic lupus erythematosus by the absence of immunoglobulins and complement in the basement membrane).
   (c) Electromyography: reduced amplitude and duration of motor unit potentials.

Dermatomyositis is an inflammatory condition of proximal muscles, accompanied by a characteristic erythematous or eczematous rash which is lilac-coloured (heliotropic) around the eyes and nailfolds. There is an association with underlying malignancy and the condition may be a feature of the connective tissue overlap syndromes.

The presenting complaint is usually due to the proximal weakness. The patient may have noticed difficulty in rising from a chair or in combing the hair. Little more than a dull ache is experienced from the affected muscles. There may be a history of dysphagia or dysarthria, as the bulbar muscles can be involved; the ocular muscles are never affected. In cases associated with underlying malignancy (most often the breast) the condition may become apparent sometime before the presentation of the neoplasm.

Prednisolone is the treatment of choice, with bed-rest during the acute episode. The reduction in dosage during convalescence should be gradual in order to prevent relapse. Conditions associated with underlying malignancy may make a dramatic recovery on removal of the tumour. Immunosuppressives and plasma exchange have been of benefit in some resistant cases.

Question 23

This patient with asthma presented with a fever and night sweats.
1. What is the most likely diagnosis?
2. What would a blood film show?
3. What is the treatment for this condition?

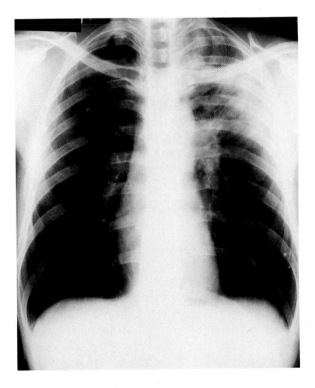

Answer to question 23

1. Cryptogenic pulmonary eosinophilia.
2. Eosinophilia.
3. Oral prednisolone.

The characteristic radiographic features of this disease are the homogeneous, ill-defined peripheral shadows which are non-segmental in distribution and predominantly affect the upper lobes. This appearance in the lungs has been described as the photographic negative of pulmonary oedema. Pulmonary eosinophilia covers those conditions which are associated with a blood eosinophilia. The classification of this group of infiltrative disorders was originally based on clinical features; it is now based on their aetiology. Identifiable causes include helminth infections, drug reactions (e.g. nitrofurantoin, sulphonamides, salazopyrine), *Aspergillus fumigatus* and other fungi. The causes of the eosinophilic infiltrations associated with the systemic vasculitides and cryptogenic pulmonary eosinophilia (20% of all cases in the UK) remain unknown.

Approximately half of all patients with cryptogenic pulmonary eosinophilia are adult asthmatics, the pulmonary eosinophilia usually occurring after the onset of asthma. The clinical features of cryptogenic pulmonary eosinophilia are severe systemic symptoms including fever and weight-loss; in addition there is usually dyspnoea and an unproductive cough. The important differential diagnosis in these patients, especially those on intermittent steroid treatment, is pulmonary tuberculosis. Typically, the IgE levels in patients with cryptogenic pulmonary eosinophilia are normal (a blood eosinophilia and raised IgE would suggest allergic bronchopulmonary aspergillosis or helminth infestation).

There is a striking improvement in the patient's condition on starting oral prednisolone. Equally dramatic is the clearing of the chest radiograph within 24 hours of starting treatment.

Question 24

1. From what condition is this patient suffering?
2. Name three extra-articular complications.

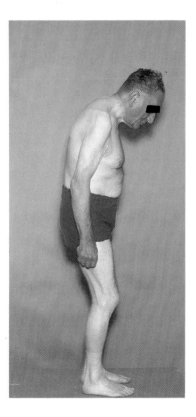

Answer to question 24

1. Ankylosing spondylitis.
2. (a) Iritis.
   (b) Aortitis.
   (c) Cardiac conduction defects (commonly first degree block).
   (d) Apical pulmonary fibrosis.
   (e) Amyloid (rare).

Ankylosing spondylitis presents in young adults with low back pain and has a male to female ratio of about 8 : 1. Of the seronegative, arthropathies this condition has the greatest association with HLA-B27 (95% of cases). As spinal fusion progresses, pain becomes less prominent and the typical deformity develops: a straight lumbar spine with thoracic kyphosis and cervical lordosis (illustrated). One-third of patients have a peripheral arthritis during the course of the disease, principally affecting the weight-bearing joints of the lower limbs. The arthropathy of psoriasis, Reiter's disease, Crohn's disease and ulcerative colitis can be identical.

Clinical examination reveals reduced spinal movements in all directions, with less than 5 cm longitudinal expansion of the lumbar spine on full flexion and an increase in the chest circumference on inspiration of less than 2.5 cm.

Indomethacin and phenylbutazone are the anti-inflammatory agents of choice for the condition, with physiotherapy, particularly in the early stages, to improve posture and minimise deformity. Severe hip disease can be managed with arthroplasty.

Question 25

This patient has chronic renal failure. He was found to have hyperuricaemia, glycosuria and aminoaciduria.
1. What does this blood film show?
2. What is the likely diagnosis?

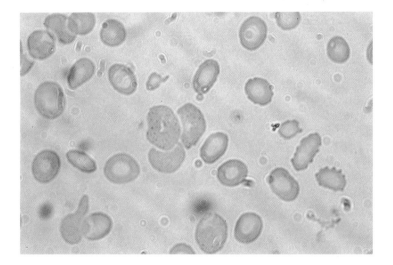

Answer to question 25

1. Punctate basophilia of red blood cells.
2. Lead nephropathy.

Basophilic stippling is not pathognomonic of lead poisoning and is seen in any severe anaemic state. For this reason patients suspected of having lead poisoning should have their blood lead levels checked and urine screened for porphyrin precursors. Coproporphyrin III is easily detected by acidifying a sample of urine with acetic acid, adding ether, and showing red fluorescence in the ether layer under a Wood's lamp. Punctate basophilia may be confused with siderocytes containing Pappenheimer bodies: these granules are larger and usually occur in pairs. The small granules responsible for basophilic stippling are small clumps of degraded RNA.

The anaemia found in lead poisoning is rarely severe and does not fully explain the striking pallor of patients with plumbism. The typical features of chronic lead poisoning (abdominal colic, blue gum lines, anaemia, peripheral neuropathy and encephalopathy) may be complicated by a tubulointerstitial nephropathy. A characteristic feature of lead nephropathy is hyperuricaemia which may cause 'saturnine gout'. ('Saturnism' is another name for lead poisoning after the reputation given by Burton (1621) to those born under the planet Saturn: 'melancholy by nature as lead and such like minerals'.)

Question 26

1. What valve is shown by this echocardiograph?
2. Describe two abnormalities.
3. What is the diagnosis?

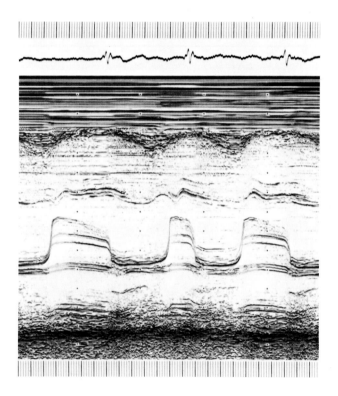

Answer to question 26

1. Mitral valve.
2. (a) Valve cusp thickening.
   (b) Reduced mid-diastolic closure rate of anterior cusp.
   (c) Anterior motion of posterior cusp during diastole.
   (d) Atrial fibrillation.
3. Mitral stenosis.

The recording is of the mitral valve; comparison with the electrocardiographic rhythm strip at the top of the trace shows the valve opening in diastole and closing in systole.

The posterior cusp however has been drawn forwards during diastole (in a normal valve the cusps should separate) because of tethering to the anterior cusp. In addition, the mid-diastolic closure rate of the anterior cusp is reduced. With a normal valve the echo from this cusp has an M-shaped pattern because of a partial closure between ventricular relaxation and atrial systole.

In mitral stenosis the ventricular filling rate is slowed, and this finding correlates better with the severity of stenosis than does the reduced mid-diastolic closure rate of the anterior cusp.

Question 27

This patient has an abnormal glucose tolerance test.
1. What is the diagnosis?
2. Name four other radiological abnormalities found in this condition.

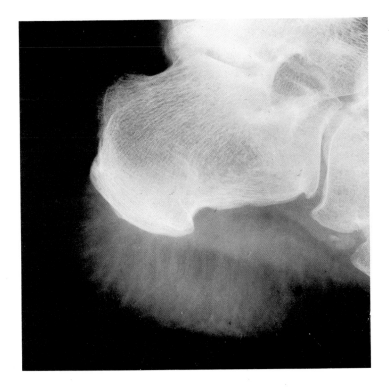

Answer to question 27

1. Acromegaly.
2. (a) Expansion of the sella turcica.
   (b) Enlarged frontal sinus.
   (c) Thickened skull vault.
   (d) Prognathous jaw.
   (e) Tufting of the terminal phalanges.
   (f) Osteoarthritis.
   (g) Chondrocalcinosis.
   (h) Visceromegaly.

Soft tissue overgrowth is a characteristic finding of acromegaly and over 90% of cases have a heel pad thickness of over 22 mm. The distance measured is from the tuberosity of the os calcis to the skin surface. Response to treatment can be monitored by serial measurements of the heel pad thickness and mapping of the visual fields.

Question 28

1. What is the diagnosis?
2. Name four appropriate investigations.

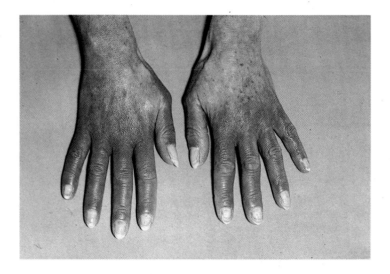

Answer to question 28

1. Raynaud's syndrome.
2. Appropriate investigations include:
   (a) Thoracic outlet radiology.
   (b) Auto-antibody screen (antinuclear antibodies, rheumatoid factor).
   (c) Erythrocyte sedimentation rate.
   (d) Cryoglobulins.
   (e) Cold agglutinins.
   (f) Protein electrophoresis.
   (g) Plasma viscosity.

The skin colour changes of Raynaud's phenomenon are the result of intense peripheral vasospasm in response to cold or emotional stimuli. Initially the extremity becomes pale, then cyanosed, and on recovery a dusky red. In cases without an underlying cause the condition is known as 'Raynaud's disease' or 'primary Raynaud's syndrome'. This is seen most commonly in young females.

A secondary Raynaud's syndrome may accompany connective tissue disease, particularly systemic sclerosis. A barium swallow demonstration of oesophageal hypomotility confirms this diagnosis. Cryoglobulinaemia, macroglobulinaemia, and cold agglutinin disease can present as Raynaud's syndrome. A cervical rib should be excluded with thoracic outlet radiology.

Question 29

What is the diagnosis?

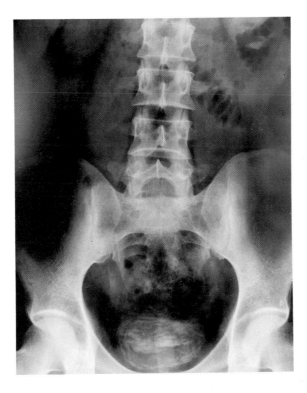

Answer to question 29

Urinary schistosomiasis.

This plain abdominal radiograph shows calcification of the bladder wall caused by *Schistosoma haematobium*. The bladder is involved in 85% of cases of urinary bilharziasis. Initially the bladder wall, although it is calcified, is not rigid and will change shape depending on the degree of bladder filling. An IVU examination may reveal filling defects in the bladder which may be due to granulomata or in chronic cases carcinoma of the bladder (this is especially common in Egypt).

Stricture and calcification of the lower ureters is also commonly seen and sometimes the whole length of the urinary tract may be affected. Schistosomiasis is an important cause of obstructive nephropathy in the Middle East, Africa and South America.

Question 30

1. What is the diagnosis?
2. Name (a) two endocrine and (b) two neurological abnormalities associated with this condition.

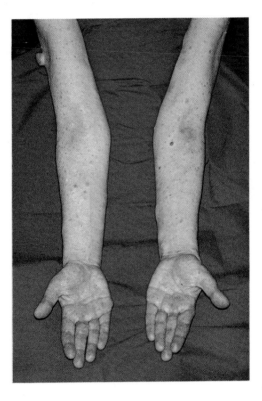

Answer to question 30

1. Neurofibromatosis (von Recklinghausen's disease).
2. (a) Endocrine:
    (i) Medullary carcinoma of thyroid.
    (ii) Phaeochromocytoma.
  (b) Neurological:
    (i) Acoustic neuroma and cranial nerve palsies.
    (ii) Spinal root tumours (with dumb-bell extension through intervertebral foramina).
    (iii) Increased incidence of glioma and meningioma.
    (iv) Obstructive hydrocephalus.

Neurofibromatosis is inherited as an autosomal dominant condition but occurs in about 50% of cases as a new mutation. Neurofibromas (local proliferations of Schwann cells and fibroblasts) and café-au-lait spots may be apparent on inspection. In addition to the endocrine and neurological complications, there may be skeletal malformations, including spina bifida, bone cysts, fibrous dysplasia and scoliosis.

Question 31

This young adult complains of pallor and listlessness.
1. What is the diagnosis?
2. Name two other radiological features of this condition.

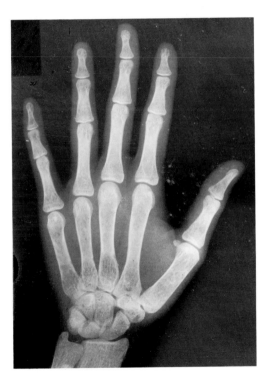

Answer to question 31

1. Thalassaemia major.
2. (a) Thickening of skull.
(b) Enlarged ribs and long bones.
(c) Paravertebral haemopoietic tissue masses.

The appearances of the metacarpals (and notably the first metacarpal) are due to marrow overactivity; evidence of marrow hyperlasia may be seen in the lesser forms and variants of thalassaemia as well as the sickle cell trait. These bone changes are much less marked than those seen in thalassaemia major, and in sickle cell disease the appearances may be modified by the presence of bone infarcts and infection.

The first changes are seen in the short bones of the extremities: expansion of bone marrow causes cortical thinning and the metacarpals and phalanges become rectangular and finally biconvex in outline. There is loss of the minor trabeculae with thickening of those that remain.

The 'hair-on-end' appearance of the skull is relatively uncommon. Hyperplasia of skull marrow will also result in poor development of the mastoids. In addition to the well-defined paravertebral mass of haemopoietic tissue, the vertebrae may show thinning with a coarse trabecular pattern, however, collapse is unusual. Hepatosplenomegaly may be noted on an abdominal radiograph.

Question 32

1. What is this condition?
2. What is the cause?
3. How should it be treated?

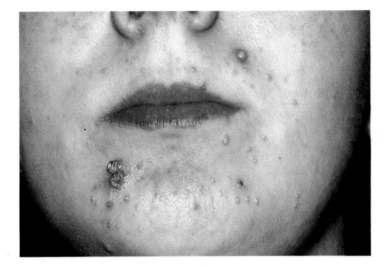

Answer to question 32

1. Molluscum contagiosum.
2. Pox virus.
3. Puncture of the lesions and application of iodine, phenol or liquid nitrogen.

Molluscum contagiosum is a condition found more frequently in children than in adults and is characterised by elevated round lesions with a central punctum, usually over the face and neck. Larger isolated lesions may be encountered in adults.

A pox virus is responsible for this condition, which is frequently acquired in public baths. The lesions resolve spontaneously within a few months, but the healing may be accelerated by treatments that irritate the underlying dermis.

Question 33

1. What is this investigation?
2. What does it show?
3. What is the differential diagnosis?

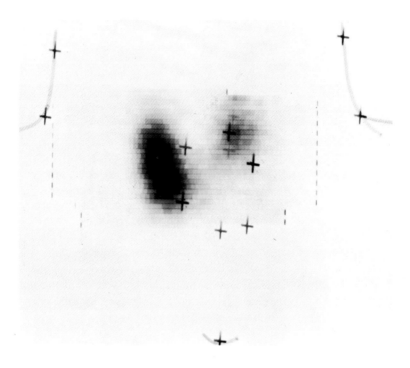

Answer to question 33

1. Radionuclide thyroid scan.
2. A solitary cold nodule.
3. (a) Adenoma.
   (b) Malignant tumour.
   (c) Localised thyroiditis.
   (d) Thyroid abscess.

The radionuclide technetium-99 m is generally used in preference to radioiodine (^{131}I) because of its shorter half-life. Its disadvantage, however, is that it gives information only about 'trapping' by the thyroid gland since it is not synthesised into thyroxine.

A thyroid scan will determine whether a nodule found on clinical examination is functioning (hot) or non-functioning (cold). A functioning nodule is almost invariably benign whereas up to 20% of solitary non-functioning nodules are malignant.

Ultrasound provides useful information in the investigation of a solitary cold nodule. Cystic lesions are easily distinguished, and since the majority are benign adenomas, these may be aspirated percutaneously and the aspirate sent for cytological examination. Conversely, if ultrasound shows the nodule to be solid, surgical excision is advisable for an accurate histological diagnosis. Some centres advocate the removal of all solitary nodules, solid or cystic, to allow the diagnosis to be made with confidence.

Question 34

1. What is this lesion?
2. Name three causes.

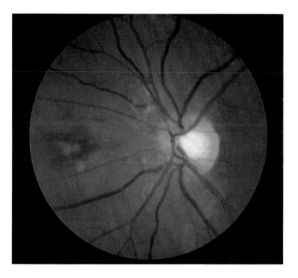

Answer to question 34

1. Roth spot.
2. (a) Infective endocarditis.
   (b) Connective tissue diseases.
   (c) Severe anaemia.

A Roth spot is an oval or boat-shaped retinal haemorrhage with a pale centre. This lesion is classically associated with infective endocarditis, but is only seen in about 5% of cases. Other signs which support a diagnosis of infective endocarditis include changing heart murmurs, cardiac failure, pyrexia, splenomegaly, systemic embolisation, haematuria, malaise and weight-loss, clubbing, splinter haemorrhages, Osler's nodes and rarely Janeway lesions.

Question 35

This patient presented with recurrent episodes of renal colic.
1. What is the diagnosis?
2. Name three causes of this condition.

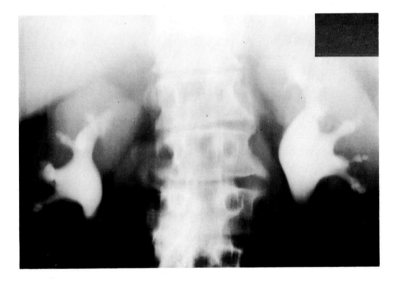

Answer to question 35

1. Renal papillary necrosis.
2. (a) Analgesic abuse.
   (b) Diabetes mellitus.
   (c) Sickle cell disease.
   Less commonly:
   (d) Acute pyelonephritis.
   (e) Ureteric obstruction.
   (f) Chronic alcoholism.
   (g) Polyarteritis nodosa.

Evidence of renal papillary necrosis may be found on a plain abdominal film when the detached papillae are seen as triangular calcific densities overlying the pelvicalyceal systems.

An IVU may show 'empty' calyces which can be confused with the clubbed calyces of chronic pyelonephritis. There may be central clefts in the papillae if the necrosis is incomplete or contrast may form a collar around the base of the papillae where they are becoming detached. The sloughed papillae may remain in the pelvicalyceal systems as filling defects.

This condition presents with renal colic, haematuria, urinary tract infections and ultimately renal failure. Papillary necrosis is probably under-diagnosed, with analgesic addiction still being the commonest cause; it is five times more common in women than in men.

Question 36

This patient developed these lesions during the course of a long illness necessitating parenteral nutrition.
What is the diagnosis?

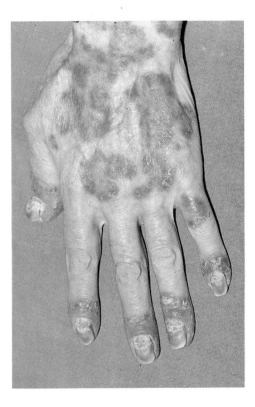

Answer to question 36

Zinc deficiency.

Zinc deficiency can arise in infants as the result of a rare autosomal recessive disorder of intestinal transport (acrodermatitis enteropathica). Similar clinical features develop in adults following several months of zinc deprivation; the condition is a recognised complication of parenteral nutrition. Psoriaform skin lesions and alopecia are typical. The lesions are elevated, erythematous and scaly and concentrated around the mouth, axillae, knuckles and perianal regions. Nail dystrophy, bloody paronychia, glossitis, stomatitis and impaired wound-healing are associated features. The patient has poor resistance to infection due to depressed leucocyte chemotaxis, and may complain of altered taste sensation (dysgeusia).

The diagnosis is confirmed by measuring the zinc concentration in hair and serum. Patients characteristically respond well to zinc therapy.

Question 37

1. What is the diagnosis?
2. Give three pulmonary complications of this condition.

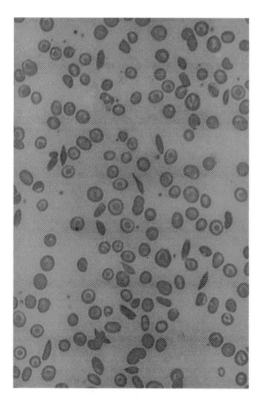

Answer to question 37

1. Sickle cell anaemia.
2. (a) Pneumonia (particularly pneumococcal).
  (b) Pulmonary infarction.
  (c) Sickle chest syndrome.
  (d) Interstitial fibrosis.
  (e) Cor pulmonale.

The blood film shows anisocytosis, poikilocytosis, sickle and target cells. The diagnosis is sickle cell anaemia and may be confirmed with haemoglobin electrophoresis. The sickle gene is present in 10% of the British Negro population.

Sickling occurs on deoxygenation. This change is initially reversible, but eventually permanent erythrocyte membrane damage occurs, leading to persistence of the sickle shape. These cells have a shortened life-span, and splenic trapping results in infarction. In acute cases a friction rub may be heard over the spleen. Subsequent splenic atrophy predisposes the patient to infection.

In treating sickle crises, exchange transfusion is preferable to simple transfusion, which causes an increase in whole blood viscosity. Recently it has been shown that a significant number of anaplastic crises are precipitated by infection with parvovirus.

The sickle chest syndrome presents with pleuritic chest pain and coughing. The physical signs and radiographic changes suggest lung consolidation, but no infectious cause is found. Recurrent attacks lead to pulmonary fibrosis and cor pulmonale.

Question 38

1. What is the likely diagnosis?
2. Which single investigation would you request to confirm this?

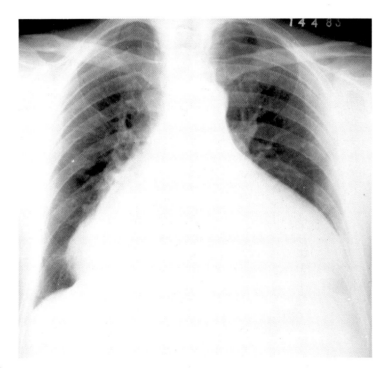

Answer to question 38

1. Pericardial effusion.
2. Echocardiogram.

The distinction between a pericardial effusion and an enlarged heart on a plain chest radiograph can rarely be made with certainty. However, a rapid increase in the cardiac diameter over a short period and a flask-shaped cardiac outline may be diagnostic. A pericardial effusion of some 150 ml may be necessary before there is any significant change in the cardiac outline.

The accuracy of echocardiography has rendered obsolete techniques such as fluoroscopy to show reduced pulsation along the cardiac border and contrast studies to show the cardiac chambers in relation to the border of the heart.

It should be remembered that a small effusion which causes barely discernible changes on a chest radiograph is capable of causing life-threatening cardiac tamponade.

Question 39

This patient has an atypical pneumonia.
1. Name the skin lesion.
2. From what condition is he suffering?
3. Name three risk factors for this condition.

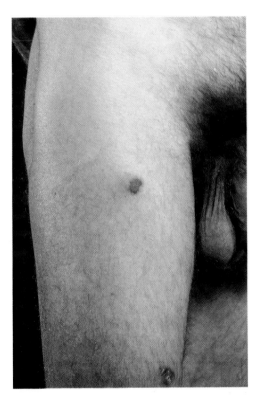

Answer to question 39

1. Kaposi's sarcoma.
2. Acquired immune deficiency syndrome.
3. (a) Homosexuality.
   (b) Intravenous drug abuse.
   (c) Haemophilia.
   (d) Blood transfusion recipient.
   (e) Haitian origin.
   Transplant patients on long-term immunosuppressive therapy commonly suffer from opportunistic infections and some may develop Kaposi's sarcoma.

The acquired immune deficiency syndrome (AIDS) is believed to be caused by the human T-cell lymphotropic virus III and has a latent period of between a few months and several years following inoculation. Cellular immunity becomes depressed with the characteristic development of a T-helper cell lymphopenia. Kaposi's sarcoma, previously a condition of elderly Ashkenazi Jews, young male Africans and Mediterranean races, commonly accompanies the syndrome.

The lesions take the form of purplish nodules, papules or plaques and consist of small vessel proliferations with clusters of pleomorphic spindle cells. Lymphadenopathy and visceral involvement are typical of the African variety and cases associated with AIDS. Patients who present with Kaposi's sarcoma alone tend to have a better prognosis than those with co-existing opportunistic infection. The condition has a 40% mortality, with most deaths occurring in the first year.

Opportunistic infections are usually due to *pneumocystis carinii*, cytomegalovirus, atypical mycobacteria, *Candida* spp. and *Nocardia* spp. *Pneumocystis* is treatable with high dose septrin and requires lung biopsy for certain diagnosis.

The transmission of AIDS seems to follow the same pattern as hepatitis B, and similar precautions should be taken in the management of suspected cases.

Question 40

This 50-year-old patient complains of low back pain. Name the three most likely diagnoses.

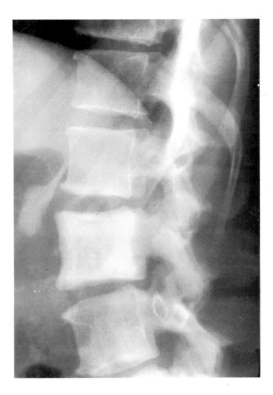

Answer to question 40

(a) Paget's disease.
(b) Malignant metastasis.
(c) Lymphoma.

The solitary dense vertebra, without evidence of destruction, is almost always caused by one of these three conditions.

Primary carcinomas of the breast or prostate are usually responsible for sclerotic bony metastases. Lymphoma is unlikely to affect a single vertebral body without clinical evidence of the disease. Pointers to the diagnosis of Paget's disease are expansion of the involved vertebra, and concentration of sclerosis around the edges of the vertebral body giving a 'picture-frame' appearance. Rarely a haemangioma causes increased density of a vertebral body; however, this is usually accompanied by vertical striations which are characteristic of this condition.

Question 41

1. What does this liver biopsy show?
2. Name five possible causes.

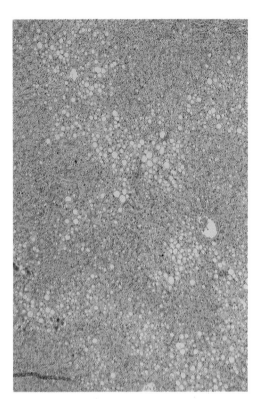

Answer to question 41

1. Fatty change.
2. (a) Alcohol.
   (b) Diabetes mellitus.
   (c) Obesity.
   (d) Starvation.
   (e) Severe infections, e.g. smallpox, septicaemia.
   (f) Pregnancy.
   (g) Drugs, e.g. methotrexate, corticosteroids, high doses of tetracycline.
   (h) Poisoning, e.g. phosphorus, carbon tetrachloride.
   (i) Cystic fibrosis.
   (j) Inflammatory bowel disease.
   (k) Reye's syndrome.

Clear vacuoles of fat within the cytoplasm are seen throughout the liver; the parenchyma is otherwise normal. Other rare causes of fatty infiltration of the liver which occur with additional histopathological changes include: (a) disseminated TB (b) Wilson's disease (c) cardiac failure (d) sickle cell disease.

Reye's syndrome is an extremely rare condition of childhood characterised by fever and vomiting, encephalopathy, hypoglycaemia, and extensive fatty infiltration of the liver, heart and proximal renal tubules. It occurs worldwide, with some clustering of cases. The aetiology is unknown, although the fact that this syndrome often follows an upper respiratory infection has lead to the suggestion that a virus might be responsible. The mortality is approximately 50%, and survivors do not show any residual liver disease. Treatment is supportive and mainly directed at controlling the cerebral oedema.

Question 42

This is the chest radiograph of a 24-year-old patient who has taken an overdose.
1. What is the abnormality?
2. Which drug most commonly causes this appearance?

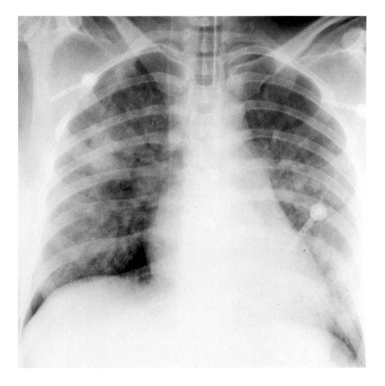

Answer to question 42

1. Pulmonary oedema.
2. Salicylate overdose.

Pulmonary oedema is a serious complication of salicylate overdose. A recent study has shown that pulmonary oedema may occur in more than a third of patients over 30 years old who have taken a significant salicylate overdose. Increased capillary permeability is thought to be the cause of pulmonary oedema; consequently there is often accompanying cerebral oedema.

Pulmonary oedema may also be precipitated or exacerbated by the over-enthusiastic use of forced alkaline diuresis. Less commonly self-poisoning with paraquat or narcotics causes pulmonary oedema.

Question 43

This patient was completely well 12 hours ago.
1. What is the diagnosis?
2. What treatment is urgently required?

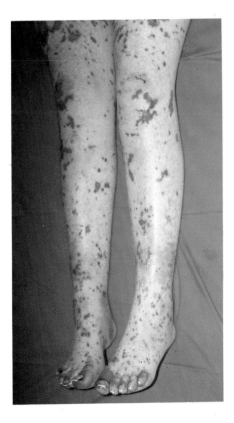

Answer to question 43

1. Meningococcal septicaemia.
2. Benzylpenicillin (chloramphenicol if the patient is allergic to penicillin).

An infrequent complication of colonisation of the nasopharynx with meningococci is acute septicaemia with rapid systemic multiplication of organisms and endotoxaemia. Within a few hours of developing an influenza-like illness with gastroenteritis, fever and tachycardia, the patient may develop circulatory collapse with haemorrhagic skin lesions and mucosal bleeding.

Meningococcal toxin is a potent cause of vascular endothelial damage with local inflammation and disseminated intravascular coagulation; vasodilation and myocardial involvement leads to shock.

Adrenal haemorrhage is a recognised feature of meningococcal septicaemia (Waterhouse-Friderichsen syndrome) but in most cases cortisol levels are appropriately elevated, and rise further following administration of ACTH. The use of corticosteroids in septicaemic shock is controversial.

Diagnosis of meningococcal septicaemia is reliably confirmed by blood culture and identification of specific antigen with immunoelectrophoresis. Penicillin should always be administered before these results become available. Rifampicin or minocycline are recommended as prophylaxis for contacts.

Question 44

This patient is 26 weeks pregnant.
1. What is the diagnosis?
2. How would you manage this patient?

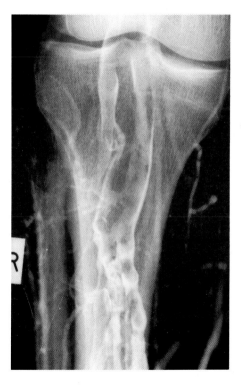

Answer to question 44

1. Deep vein thrombosis.
2. (a) Heparin infusion for 10 days.
  (b) Subcutaneous heparin until term.
  (c) Prophylactic subcutaneous heparin for 6 weeks after labour.

The deep veins show extensive clot with 'tramlines' of contrast on either side of the central filling defect. Warfarin should never be used in the first trimester of pregnancy, because of its teratogenicity. An intravenous heparin infusion should be commenced as soon as the diagnosis is made. After 10 days, subcutaneous heparin twice daily should be started. The heparin dose needed to maintain a satisfactory activated partial thromboplastin time increases as pregnancy progresses. If self-injection is unacceptable, warfarin may be used providing it is not given before the 12th week of pregnancy. At the onset of labour heparin should be stopped. It is generally recommended that anti-coagulation should be continued throughout the 6 weeks of the puerperium.

Question 45

This is the blood film of a patient with a family history of gall stones.
1. What is the diagnosis?
2. What test will help to confirm this?
3. What treatment is required?

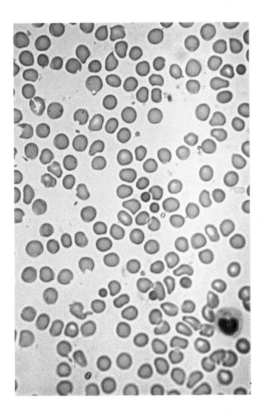

Answer to question 45

1. Hereditary spherocytosis.
2. Increased red cell osmotic fragility.
3. Splenectomy.

Hereditary spherocytosis is a Mendelian dominant disorder of erythrocytes resulting in abnormal membrane permeability to sodium. In this condition spherocytes are identified in the peripheral blood as small round cells without central pallor. The number of spherocytes seen in a blood film is extremely variable. There may also be anaemia, a 5–20% reticulocytosis and occasionally normoblasts.

The spleen is almost always enlarged, and trapping of abnormal cells leads to acholuric jaundice. Pigment gall stones occur in 50% of cases. Other complications include leg ulceration, haemolytic and aplastic crises.

Splenectomy is indicated in all but the mildest of cases, and results in cessation of haemolysis, resolution of jaundice and decreased incidence of gall stones and aplastic crises.

Question 46

This is the barium meal of a 69-year-old woman.
1. What is the radiological abnormality?
2. What is the likely cause?

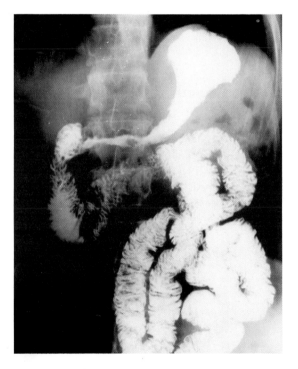

Answer to question 46

1. Small, irregular stomach.
2. Gastric carcinoma (linitis plastica).

Extensive submucosal infiltration by tumour results in the characteristic appearance on barium examination of a small, rigid stomach.

Although primary gastric carcinoma is by far the commonest cause, a similar picture may be seen in the following conditions:

(i) Post-irradiation.
(ii) Corrosive gastritis.
(iii) Lymphoma.
(iv) Crohn's disease.
(v) Metastatic disease, e.g. carcinoma of the pancreas.

Question 47

1. What is the diagnosis?
2. Name three causes.
3. Give one test that will confirm the abnormality.

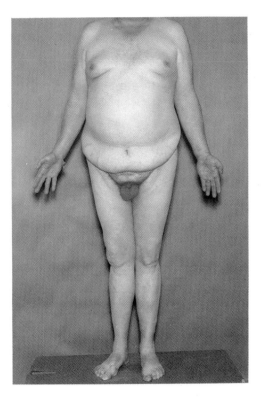

Answer to question 47

1. Cushing's syndrome.
2. (a) Iatrogenic.
   (b) Cushing's disease (increased pituitary ACTH).
   (c) Adrenal adenoma or carcinoma.
   (d) Ectopic ACTH production from benign tumours.
       (Ectopic ACTH from a malignant tumour is unlikely, as these patients are usually cachectic and the diagnosis is a chance biochemical finding.)
   (e) Pseudocushing's syndrome of alcoholism.
3. (a) Dexamethasone suppression test.
   (b) 24-hour urinary free cortisol.

The truncal obesity, peripheral wasting and abdominal striae are typical of a patient suffering from Cushing's syndrome; echymoses, hirsutes, hypertension, osteoporosis, moon face and a buffalo hump may be other findings. Metabolic consequences of the condition include hypokalaemic alkalosis, glucose intolerance and hyperlipidaemia.

Iatrogenic disease is common. Most other cases are due to increased ACTH production from a pituitary macro- or microadenoma (Cushing's disease). Adrenal tumours are less frequently discovered and the carcinomas tend to be androgen-producing.

Cushing's syndrome is suggested by loss of diurnal plasma variation and increased 24-hour urinary excretion of cortisol. The administration of glucocorticoid towards the end of the day is a particularly potent stimulus to pituitary-adrenal axis suppression and forms the basis of the overnight dexamethasone suppression test. Pituitary and adrenal tumours are barely influenced by this (dexamethasone does not interfere with cortisol assay) and in such cases morning cortisol levels remain elevated.

The distinction between adrenal and pituitary aetiologies may be established following further administration of dexamethasone, which tends to suppress the pituitary adenomas. The availability of ACTH assay and CAT scanning has greatly simplified this distinction.

Question 48

This Indian man had ulcers on his lower legs.
1. What is the diagnosis?
2. What is the treatment?

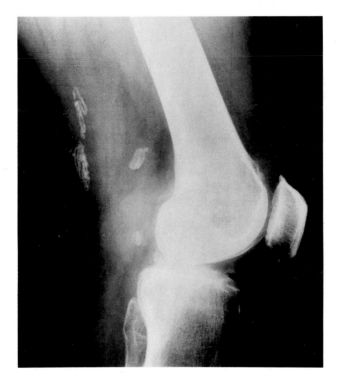

Answer to question 48

1. Guinea-worm disease (dracontiasis).
2. (a) Extraction of the guinea-worm.
   (b) A nitroimidazole (e.g. niridazole or metronidazole).
   (c) Tetanus toxoid injection.

Dracontiasis is very common in West Africa and India. Transmission is by drinking water containing the larvae of *Dracunculus medinensis*, which are carried by water fleas. After ingestion the female migrates to the skin, usually of the lower limbs. An ulcer forms and when the protruding worm is in contact with water, larvae are released. Infection of the ulcer with tetanus bacillus is a frequent complication.

The guinea-worm is one of the largest nematodes, and may reach a length of 50 cm. Extraction is most elegantly achieved by slowly winding the worm around a match-stick. Calcification, which gives the diagnostic radiological appearance, occurs only after death of the guinea-worm.

Question 49

What has happened?

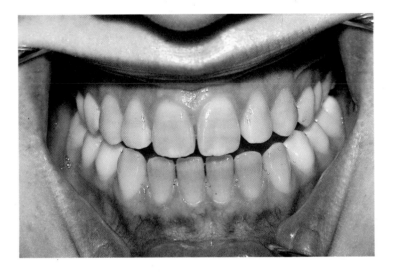

Answer to question 49

This patient has been given tetracycline in childhood. The drug is bound by calcium and may become deposited in growing bones and teeth. It should not be given to pregnant women or children under the age of twelve, as dental discoloration or hypoplasia may result. The affinity of tetracycline for calcium results in reduced absorption if this drug is given with milk.

Question 50

This patient presented with painful eyes and joints.
1. What is the likely diagnosis?
2. Name two tests that will help to confirm this.

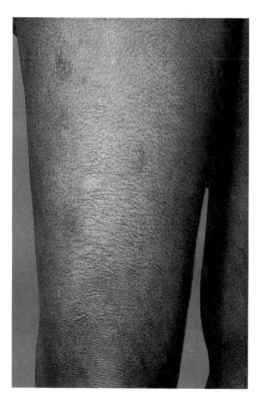

Answer to question 50

1. Sarcoidosis.
2. (a) Biopsy from skin or lymph node demonstrating non-caseating epithelioid granulomas.
   (b) Positive Kveim test – appearance of granulomas at the site of an intradermal injection of human sarcoid tissue.
   (c) Elevation of serum angiotensin converting enzyme.

Abnormalities on respiratory function testing, a negative tuberculin test and hypercalcaemia are features of sarcoidosis, but less helpful in establishing the diagnosis. Changes on the chest radiograph (bilateral hilar lymphadenopathy with or without pulmonary infiltrates) are associated with erythema nodosum and an acute onset and tend not to be features of cutaneous sarcoid. This condition is characterised by lupus pernio, scar infiltration or a diffuse plaque form that is more common in Negroes; the lesions are concentrated over the shoulders, buttocks and thighs (illustrated). Bone cysts, particularly in the phalanges and metacarpals, often accompany these manifestations.

The hypercalcaemia of sarcoidosis is similar to that of hypervitaminosis D. The serum phosphate is in the normal range and there is a moderate hypercalciuria. Patients may have symptoms from hypercalcaemia, but respond well to steroid suppression.

Lung function abnormalities consist of a restrictive ventilatory defect with reduced transfer factor. Changes in the T-lymphocyte subpopulations lead to a deficiency in the expression of delayed hypersensitivity and probably account for the negative tuberculin test in those previously positive.

An acute onset with erythema nodosum and hilar lymphadenopathy carries a good prognosis and little treatment is required. Corticosteroids are reserved for cases with severe uveitis, hypercalcaemia and exertional dyspnoea. In this last group there is no evidence that steroids modify the course of the disease.

Question 51

1. What is the abnormality?
2. Name three conditions in which this occurs.

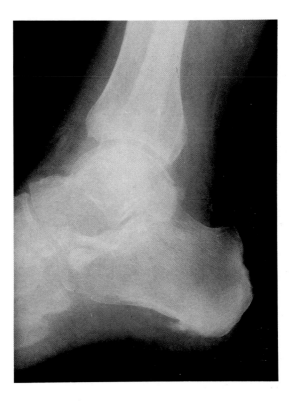

Answer to question 51

1. Calcaneal spur.
2. (a) Reiter's disease.
   (b) Psoriatic arthritis.
   (c) Rheumatoid arthritis.
   (d) Ankylosing spondylitis (rare).

The spur seen on the plantar surface of the os calcis in chronic cases of Reiter's disease has an irregular margin and may also be seen on the posterior aspect of the os calcis at the insertion of the Achilles tendon. This periosteal new bone formation results from long-standing plantar fasciitis. Well-defined calcaneal spurs may occur in otherwise normal individuals, especially young children.

Question 52

This is the blood film of a 6-year-old child.
1. What is the diagnosis?
2. Name four known predisposing factors for this condition.

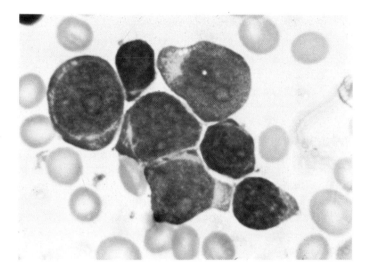

Answer to question 52

1. Acute lymphoblastic leukaemia.
2. (a) Ionising radiation.
   (b) Down's syndrome.
   (c) Benzene.
   (d) Fanconi's aplastic anaemia.
   (e) Other rare conditions caused by chromosome damage, e.g. Bloom's syndrome, Patau syndrome.
   (f) Some immunodeficiency states, e.g. ataxia-telangiectasia, sex-linked agammaglobulinaemia, Wiskott-Aldrich syndrome.

The primitive leukaemic cells in the blood film are lymphoblasts. The high nuclear to cytoplasmic ratio gives an indication of their immaturity. Acute lymphoblastic leukaemia (ALL) has increased incidence in two age-groups: it is the commonest leukaemia in children under 5 years; after the age of 55 years the incidence of ALL rises steeply.

There have been occasional case reports of acute leukaemia following the use of certain drugs (phenylbutazone and chloramphenicol) and combined chemo- and radiotheraphy.

Question 53

This is the lateral chest radiograph of a 45-year-old smoker.
What is the most likely diagnosis?

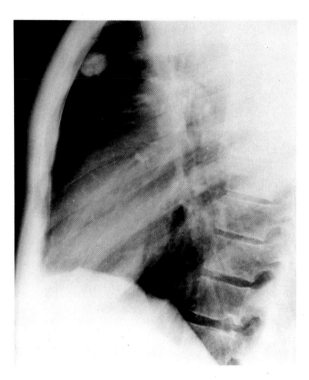

Answer to question 53

Hamartoma.

The single lung nodule is a common diagnostic problem. In the UK the differential diagnosis would include (a) primary bronchogenic carcinoma (b) bronchial adenoma (c) hamartoma (or other benign lung tumour) (d) infective granuloma (e.g. TB) (e) solitary metastasis (f) rheumatoid nodule (g) lung abscess.

Radiographic pointers to the diagnosis of hamartoma include:

(a) No change in size on serial radiographs.
(b) The outline of a hamartoma is usually clearly demarcated and is often a perfect sphere whereas carcinomas are generally ill-defined with an infiltrating edge.
(c) Hamartomas are usually less than 6 cm in diameter and a shadow larger than this is more likely to be a primary carcinoma or lung abscess.
(d) Calcification within the lesion virtually rules out a primary carcinoma, especially if it is marked and is of the 'popcorn' configuration (seen in 30% of hamartomas). Tomography will detect minor calcification and also confirm that the calcification is within the mass.
(e) Cavitation is not seen in hamartomas and indicates either a lung abscess, a primary carcinoma (usually squamous) or, rarely, a metastasis.

The differentiation between a hamartoma and a bronchial carcinoma may still be difficult and in these cases biopsy for histological examination is required.

Question 54

This patient presented with convulsions and was found to be mentally subnormal.
1. What is the diagnosis?
2. Name two tests which confirm this.

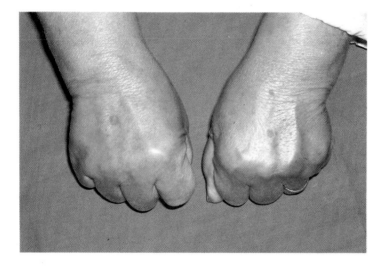

Answer to question 54

1. Pseudohypoparathyroidism.
2. (a) Low corrected calcium and high serum phosphate in the presence of normal renal function.
  (b) Appropriately elevated serum PTH (parathormone) levels.
  (c) Absence of phosphaturic response to PTH infusion.

The combination of a low serum calcium and a high serum phosphate in the presence of normal renal function is the hallmark of hypoparathyroidism. Such patients may present with convulsive seizures, tetany, metastatic calcification (e.g. the skin and basal ganglia) and cataracts. The finding of appropriately elevated serum PTH suggests an end-organ resistance to the hormone; this condition is known as 'pseudohypoparathyroidism'. Associated skeletal malformations include short stature, round face, short neck and shortening of the metacarpal and metatarsal bones – usually the 4th or 5th (illustrated). The inheritance in most families is X-linked dominant. 'Pseudopseudohypopara-thyroidism' denotes the condition of other family members with similar skeletal malformations but normal biochemistry. Patients with pseudohypoparathyroidism have an increased incidence of diabetes mellitus, hypothyroidism and gonadal dysgenesis with amenorrhoea; some hypothyroid cases have an isolated TSH deficiency.

There are several different patterns of end-organ resistance in pseudohypoparathyroidism. Type I patients, with abnormal membrane bound adenylcyclase, fail to increase urinary phosphate or cAMP following a PTH infusion. Type II patients develop an increased urinary cAMP without a phosphaturic effect and this is presumed to represent a phosphate and calcium membrane transport defect. In some patients different target organs have differing sensitivities – indeed some patients may develop osteitis fibrosa. Treatment for all cases is with vitamin D and calcium supplements.

Question 55

1. What is the diagnosis?
2. How might this patient present?

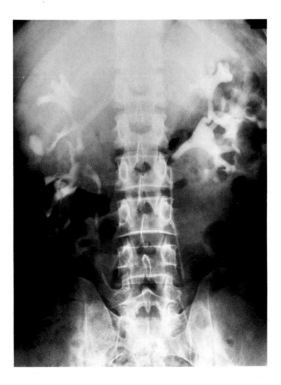

Answer to question 55

1. Polycystic disease of the kidneys.
2. (a) Abdominal pain or mass.
    (b) Haematuria.
    (c) Chronic renal failure.
    (d) Hypertension.
    (e) Urinary tract infection.

The kidneys have the distinctive appearances of polycystic disease. Both kidneys are large and the pelvicalyceal systems are distorted by innumerable cysts; these are best seen in the nephrogram phase of an IVU. In advanced cases the calyces are deformed to give a 'spider's leg' appearance. It should be remembered that the kidneys in adult polycystic disease may not be enlarged; furthermore the disease may be asymmetrical and occasionally the pyelogram is entirely normal. If there is any doubt ultrasound will clarify the diagnosis and angiography is now rarely indicated.

Patients with adult polycystic disease usually present between the ages of 35 and 45 years with one of the features listed above. Less common complications include:

(a) Polycythaemia.
(b) Obstructive uropathy (due to large medial lower pole cysts).
(c) Renal lithiasis.

Question 56

This is the Vitalograph trace of a 28-year-old man who complains of shortness of breath and 'wheeze'.

FEV_1 = 2600 ml
FVC = 4400 ml
FEV_1/FVC = 60%
PEFR = 156 l/min

1. Describe the respiratory defect.
2. What response would you predict with bronchodilator therapy?

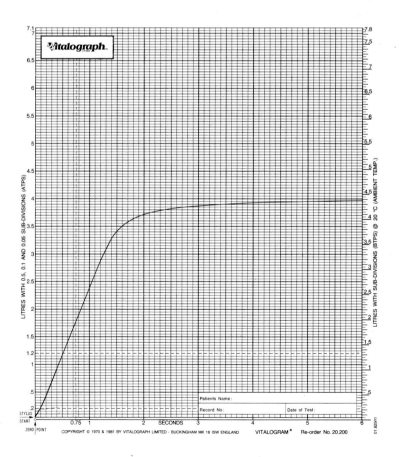

Answer to question 56

1. Obstructive defect.
2. None; the Vitalograph trace demonstrates an upper airways obstruction that would not respond to bronchodilator therapy. The 'wheeze' described by the patient was stridor!

An FEV_1/FVC ratio of less than 75% in a patient of this age is abnormal and characteristic of an obstructive ventilatory defect. The PEFR in this case is disproportionately low and the typical smooth curve of the Vitalograph trace has been lost. The straight initial upstroke gives the diagnosis – large airways obstruction (e.g. retrosternal thyroid, tracheal stricture following tracheotomy).

In cases of significant upper airway obstruction the FEV_1/PEFR ratio is greater than 10; in this case it is 16.7. A flow volume loop would have a characteristic rectangular appearance.

Question 57

1. What is the radiological abnormality?
2. What is the likely diagnosis?
3. Name three other clinical features of this condition.

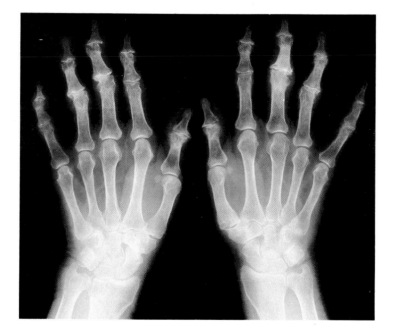

Answer to question 57

1. An erosive arthropathy involving the distal and proximal interphalangeal joints.
2. Psoriatic arthritis.
3. (a) Psoriasis.
   (b) Nail pitting and ridging, onycholysis.
   (c) Anterior uveitis.
   (d) Keratoconjunctivitis sicca.
   (e) Aortic incompetence.

Psoriatic arthritis is not uncommon; the incidence in the general population is 1 in 1000. It occurs in approximately 12% of patients with psoriasis. Rarely psoriatic arthritis occurs before the skin manifestations.

There are five clinical patterns of psoriatic arthritis:

1. Asymmetrical distal interphalangeal joint involvement.
2. Symmetrical arthritis indistinguishable from rheumatoid arthritis but persistently seronegative.
3. Arthritis mutilans, with telescoping of digits and extensive bone resorption.
4. Asymmetrical oligarthritis or monarthritis.
5. Sacroiliitis and spondylitis with or without any of the other patterns of peripheral joint involvement.

Question 58

This confused patient has a gastrointestinal disturbance.
What is the underlying disorder?

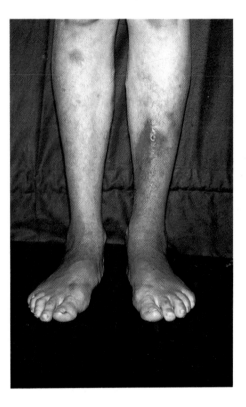

Answer to question 58

Pellagra.

Pellagra occurs as a result of nicotinic acid deficiency. The condition is often associated with protein and other vitamin deficiencies and is common in parts of the world where maize products are a principal source of food. Maize is rich in nicotinic acid that is biologically unavailable. In the Western world chronic alcoholism is the commonest cause of nicotinic acid deficiency.

Initially the patient complains of loss of appetite with a change in bowel habit, weakness, insomnia and glossitis. Skin lesions are at first erythematous and pruritic but vesiculation and peeling leaves a dirty brown discolouration which may be almost black in dark-skinned patients. This discoloration is most prominent over exposed body areas, particularly the face and dorsum of the hands and feet (illustrated).

The neurological features comprise nervousness, confusion, tremor, reduced reflexes and painful hands and feet. With the administration of folic acid, riboflavine, thiamine and cyanocobalamin some of the symptoms and signs may be alleviated which suggests that the full-blown condition arises as a result of a multi-vitamin deficiency.

Tryptophan is a biochemical precursor of nicotinic acid and a similar clinical picture has been described with Hartnup disease (impaired intestinal absorption and renal wasting of tryptophan), malignant carcinoid syndrome (diversion of tryptophan to 5HT) and with isoniazid therapy (the conversion of tryptophan to nicotinic acid is pyridoxine-dependent).

Question 59

1. What is this investigation?
2. What does it show?

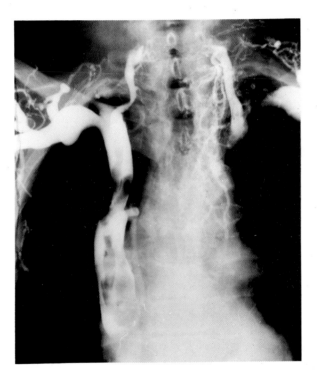

Answer to question 59

1. Superior vena cavogram.
2. Clot in the superior vena cava with collateral circulation.

The technique of superior vena cavography involves the rapid venous injection of contrast into both arms. Sequential films demonstrate the subclavian veins and superior vena cava (SVC). The indications for superior vena cavography are:

(a) Upper limb engorgement thought to be due to venous obstruction.
(b) SVC obstruction – usually due to carcinoma of the bronchus with lymph node involvement; sometimes seen in tuberculosis and fibrosing mediastinitis.

This patient had a hypernephroma and was on prolonged bed-rest. Isolated thrombosis of the SVC is uncommon and the predisposing causes of venous thrombosis are not necessarily present.

Question 60

1. What is the diagnosis?
2. What complication of treatment can occur?
3. How is this risk minimised?

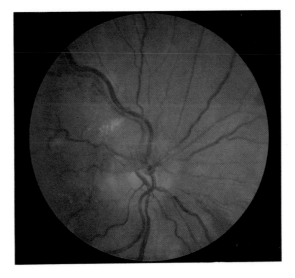

Answer to question 60

1. Malignant hypertension.
2. Cerebral infarction (often causing blindness).
3. Gradual reduction of blood pressure.

The Keith-Wagener classification of hypertensive retinopathy defines four grades of increasing severity. Grade 3 is characterised by flame-shaped haemorrhages, cotton-wool spots (retinal infarcts) and hard exudates (cholesterol deposits). The additional presence of papilloedema denotes grade 4. The outlook is equally severe in both of these groups and the term 'malignant hypertension' may be applied to either. Fibrinoid arteriolar necrosis is the characteristic histopathological finding. Before the days of effective anti-hypertensive therapy, death as a result of renal failure, myocardial infarction or stroke would usually follow within a year.

Tissue infarction may be precipitated by too rapid a reduction in blood pressure and the safest management is with bed rest and oral antihypertensives. Life-threatening cardiac failure or encephalopathy require parenteral medication.

Question 61

This is the cervical spine radiograph of a 30-year-old patient. What is the diagnosis?

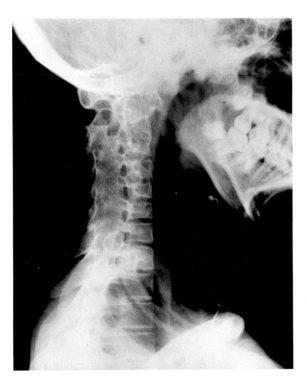

Answer to question 61

Still's disease (juvenile rheumatoid arthritis).

The striking feature of this radiograph is fusion of the posterior elements of the cervical spine and ankylosis of the apophyseal joints. Unlike adult rheumatoid arthritis, cervical spine changes are commonly seen in Still's disease, including subluxation of C1 on C2. It should be noted that there is micrognathia and the vertebral bodies are very small in view of the patient's age: this implies that there was cessation of growth in childhood (due to the inflammatory process). For this reason ankylosing spondylitis can be excluded from the differential diagnosis.

There are many other causes of vertebral fusion, including the congenital Klippel-Feil syndrome in which two or more vertebral bodies and sometimes the posterior elements are fused. The result of this 'block vertebra' is a short neck with a low hair-line and restricted neck movements.

Question 62

This patient complains of weak legs.
1. What is the abnormality?
2. Name four causes.

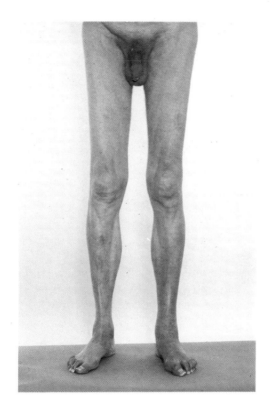

Answer to question 62

1. Proximal muscle wasting.
2. Recognised causes of proximal muscle wasting include:
   (a) Neuropathies and neuromuscular disorders
       (i) Guillain-Barré syndrome
       (ii) Eaton-Lambert syndrome
       (iii) Sarcoidosis
       (iv) Diabetic amyotrophy
   (b) Myopathies
       (i) Endocrine
           — Cushing's syndrome (often iatrogenic)
           — Thyrotoxicosis
           — Hyperparathyroidism
           — Acromegaly
           — Nelson's syndrome
       (ii) Inflammatory
           — Polymyositis
       (iii) Others
           — Alcoholism
           — Osteomalacia
           — Carcinoma
   (c) Dystrophies
       (i) Duchenne – young patients only with pseudohypertrophy of calves
       (ii) Becker – with pseudohypertrophy of calves
       (iii) Limb girdle.

Question 63

This is the chest radiograph of a 71-year-old patient who is known to have polycythaemia rubra vera.
What is the abnormal radiological sign?

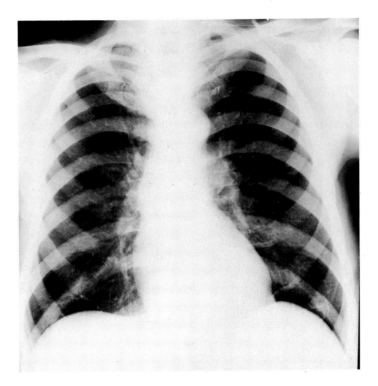

Answer to question 63

Increased bone density due to myelofibrosis.

It has been estimated that approximately half of patients with myelofibrosis previously had polycythaemia rubra vera. Unlike the development of acute myeloblastic leukaemia in patients with polycythaemia rubra vera, the onset of myelofibrosis is not thought to be related to the use of radioactive phosphorus or cytotoxic drugs.

The increased bone density occurs when there is new bone formation; translucencies may remain if fibrotic areas persist. There is corroborative evidence of myelofibrosis in this chest radiograph: the gastric air bubble is absent and the left hemidiaphragm is raised by the enlarged spleen.

Other causes of a generalised increase in bone density are:

(a) Congenital sclerosing dysplasias, e.g. osteopetrosis.
(b) Diffuse sclerotic metastases.
(c) Fluorosis.
(d) Vitamin A poisoning.
(e) Systemic mastocytosis.

Question 64

What is the diagnosis in this patient who has become acutely confused 24 hours after a road traffic accident?

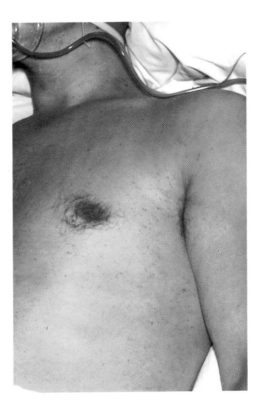

Answer to question 64

Fat embolism.

This condition occurs 12–36 hours after major fractures, but may be associated with trauma to adipose tissue or a fatty liver. It is characterised by a sudden deterioration in the neurological and cardiopulmonary condition of the patient; delirium, coma, pyrexia and respiratory distress are typical features.

The systemic release of free fatty acids causes a vasculitis and microscopic fibrin-platelet aggregation. A petechial rash may be found over the trunk (illustrated).

Treatment is mainly supportive. The adult respiratory distress syndrome is managed by providing an increased inspiratory oxygen concentration, or positive end-expiratory pressure ventilation. The benefit of corticosteroids in this condition remains unproven.

Question 65

1. Name the arrowed structures.
2. What abnormality does this ultrasound scan show?

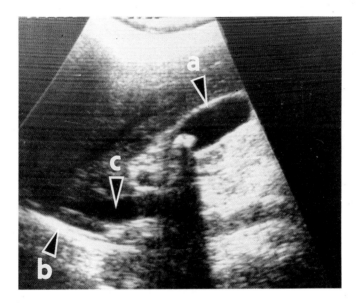

Answer to question 65

1. (a) Gall bladder.
   (b) Diaphragm.
   (c) Inferior vena cava.
2. Gall-stone.

Gall-stones are easily demonstrated by ultrasound; they are seen as highly echogenic foci which cast an acoustic shadow. The accuracy of ultrasonography in the diagnosis of cholelithiasis is claimed to be in excess of 95%. The advantage that ultrasonography of the gall bladder has over the oral cholecystogram is that it can be performed as an emergency procedure even in the presence of jaundice.

Question 66

These are the hands of a patient who presented with general malaise and weight loss accompanied by episodes of abdominal pain.
1. What is the likely diagnosis?
2. How is this confirmed?
3. What treatment is required?

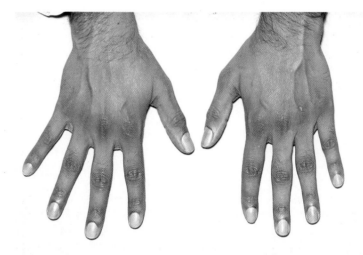

Answer to question 66

1. Primary hypoadrenalism (Addison's disease).
2. 'Synacthen test' — failure of plasma cortisol to rise following intramuscular administration of synthetic ACTH.
3. Replacement glucocorticoid and mineralocorticoid.

Increased pigmentation, particularly in scars, skin folds and the buccal mucosa, with a history of weight-loss and abdominal pain is typical of Addison's disease. Melanocyte stimulation by high levels of ACTH (and perhaps beta-MSH) serves to distinguish primary from secondary hypoadrenalism. Postural hypotension is a reliable indicator of chronic adrenal insufficiency; shock with diarrhoea and vomiting may be an extreme presentation (Addisonian crisis).

Usual laboratory findings include a slight elevation in the blood urea with hyponatraemia and hyperkalaemia. Hypoglycaemia is more characteristic of hypopituitarism because of the associated deficiency in growth hormone.

Since the decline of tuberculosis, auto-immunity has become the commonest cause of the disease. Associations include diabetes mellitus, hypothyroidism, hypoparathyroidism, pernicious anaemia and ovarian failure. Other aetiologies include metastatic carcinoma, amyloid and infarction.

In primary adrenal failure, replacement with both glucocorticoid and mineralocorticoid is required. Hydrocortisone has both properties and should be given as a twice-daily dose approximating to the circadian rhythm. Fludrocortisone (a potent mineralocorticoid) may be added if postural hypotension persists or the plasma renin fails to return to the normal range. Prednisolone has little mineralocorticoid activity and is not suitable for use as a single agent.

Question 67

This is the jejunal biopsy of a patient with progressive weight loss and arthralgia.
1. What is the diagnosis?
2. How would you treat this patient?

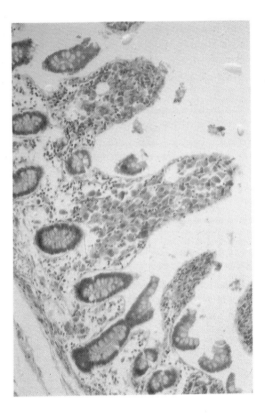

Answer to question 67

1. Whipple's disease.
2. Penicillin and streptomycin followed by tetracycline.

The columnar epithelial lining of the villi is normal but the cores of the villi are stuffed with foamy macrophages which have greyish cytoplasm. On staining with periodic acid-Schiff reagent, vivid magenta granules are seen within the cytoplasm. On electron microscopy these granules resemble rod-shaped bacilli.

This rare condition usually occurs in white, middle-aged males. The clinical features include: (a) weight loss and diarrhoea over a long period (b) abdominal pain (c) fever (d) arthralgia of large joints (e) lymphadenopathy (f) increased skin pigmentation (g) central nervous system involvement (h) purpura.

Without treatment this condition is almost invariably fatal. Treatment consists of a combination of antibiotics, usually streptomycin and penicillin for one month followed by tetracycline for one year. The response to treatment should be monitored with follow-up small intestine biopsies; the presence or absence of the macrophage inclusion bodies is the most important gauge of response. The histology of the jejunal mucosa may remain permanently abnormal despite treatment.

Question 68

1. What is this lesion?
2. How is it treated?

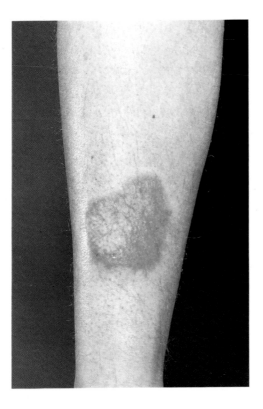

Answer to question 68

1. Necrobiosis lipoidica.
2. Protection against trauma, intralesional injection of triamcinolone.

Necrobiosis lipoidica is a condition frequently associated with diabetes mellitus. Lesions are commonest on the lower limb, particularly the shins, and may occur in the absence of diabetes or pre-date its onset. The earliest forms are red and papular; they later develop into plaques with a smooth shiny surface and a yellow telangiectatic central depression. Ulceration is a late feature.

The severity of the condition is unrelated to the quality of diabetic control, and protection against trauma is the principle of management. Some improvement may be gained from intralesional injection of triamcinolone in severe cases.

Question 69

This patient has arthritis.
1. What are the two radiological abnormalities?
2. What is the diagnosis?
3. Name three other pulmonary manifestations of this condition.

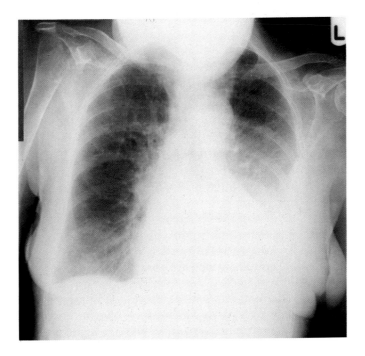

Answer to question 69

1. (a) Rheumatoid arthritis of the right shoulder.
   (b) Pleural effusion of the left lung.
2. Rheumatoid arthritis.
3. (a) Rheumatoid nodules.
   (b) Caplan's syndrome.
   (c) Fibrosing alveolitis.
   (d) Obliterative bronchiolitis.

Pleural effusions are commoner in male patients (up to 30%) with rheumatoid arthritis and are sometimes the first sign of the disease. The pleural effusion characteristically has a high protein content, a low glucose level and a high lymphocyte count; multinucleated giant cells are frequently found in these effusions. A pleural biopsy may show the typical granuloma formation. Although rheumatoid factor is usually found in rheumatoid effusions, this cannot be relied upon as diagnostic since it is often present in effusions associated with other conditions.

Lung function tests are abnormal in up to 25% of patients with rheumatoid arthritis before there is any clinical or radiological evidence of pulmonary involvement.

Pulmonary complications are commoner in seropositive patients. Pulmonary rheumatoid nodules are rarely larger than 3 cm in diameter and may be single or multiple. They occur in the lung periphery and may cavitate and then resolve. If the patient has an underlying pneumoconiosis, larger nodules may be accompanied by fibrotic reactions: this is Caplan's syndrome. Diffuse pulmonary fibrosis, indistinguishable from fibrosing alveolitis, is initially seen as basal changes which may remain static for years or progress during acute exacerbations of rheumatoid arthritis to a honeycomb lung and respiratory failure.

Penicillamine has been implicated in the aetiology of obliterative bronchiolitis. In this rare complication there is progressive obstruction of the bronchioles. There are no diagnostic radiographic changes and respiratory failure rapidly supervenes.

Question 70

1. What is the likely diagnosis in this normotensive man who, without endocrine abnormality, complains of lethargy, morning headache, and hypersomnolence?
2. How may this be confirmed?

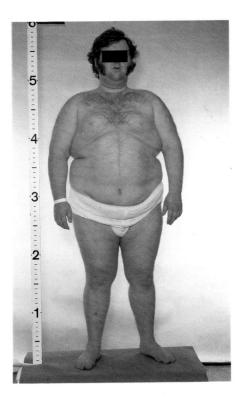

Answer to question 70

1. Sleep apnoea.
2. Sleep breathing study.

Sleep apnoea has been defined as five or more episodes during each hour of sleep in which there is a cessation of airflow at the nose and mouth lasting for at least 10 seconds. It is central if during an attack there are no detectable chest or abdominal wall movements, and obstructive if there is no airflow at the pharynx or larynx despite increased respiratory effort. Some patients may suffer from a mixed disorder. In a sleep breathing study hypoventilation can be confirmed with an earlobe oximeter by demonstrating a fall in oxygen saturation of 4–10% during apnoeic episodes.

Obstructive sleep apnoea is a recognised complication of obesity due to nocturnal pharyngeal obstruction. Intellectual deterioration occurs as a result of both nocturnal hypoxia and lack of sleep. Daytime lethargy, morning headache and personality changes may follow. The Pickwickian label is reserved for those with hypersomnolence and daytime hypoxia with a secondary polycythaemia and cor pulmonale.

A reduction in weight may relieve obesity-related obstructive apnoea. Other causes of upper airway abnormality may require surgical correction, and rarely a tracheostomy. The respiratory stimulant medroxyprogesterone has helped some patients with central sleep apnoea.

Question 71

1. What is this investigation?
2. What is the likely diagnosis?
3. Name three ways in which this condition may present.

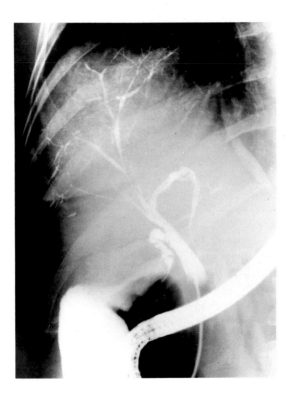

Answer to question 71

1. Endoscopic retrograde cholangiopancreatogram (ERCP).
2. Sclerosing cholangitis.
3. (a) Symptoms of intermittent obstructive jaundice.
   (b) Acute cholecystitis with abdominal pain.
   (c) Secondary biliary cirrhosis.
   (d) Hepatic failure.

In primary sclerosing cholangitis there is a progressive fibrotic and obliterative process affecting both the intra- and extrahepatic bile ducts. This leads to the characteristic beading, particularly of intrahepatic ducts, seen on ERCP.

This condition may occur in isolation or may be associated with inflammatory bowel disease (ulcerative colitis more commonly than Crohn's disease); rarely there is an association with retroperitoneal fibrosis. Secondary sclerosing cholangitis is the result of biliary surgery or cholelithiasis.

ERCP is probably the investigation of choice, and when the diagnosis is made, the possibility of associated inflammatory bowel disease should be considered.

Corticosteroids and immunosuppressive therapy have not been shown to alter the course of the disease. Antibiotics are used when infective cholangitis supervenes, and cholestyramine may be used to control pruritus. Biliary stenting has been used in cases complicated by extrahepatic obstruction. Colectomy in patients with inflammatory bowel disease has not reliably been shown to cause remission of sclerosing cholangitis.

The prognosis is poor, whatever the therapeutic manoeuvres, the mean survival after diagnosis being between 4 and 10 years.

Question 72

1. What is the abnormality?
2. Name four causes.

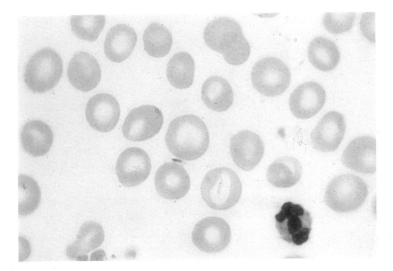

Answer to question 72

1. Macrocytosis.
2. The macrocytoses can be considered in two groups:
   (a) Megaloblastic marrow
      (i) Vitamin B_{12} deficiency
         — Addisonian pernicious anaemia
         — Post-gastrectomy
         — Structural intestinal abnormalities
         — Fish tape-worm
      (ii) Folate deficiency
         — Nutritional
         — Sprue, coeliac disease
         — Alcoholism
         — Chronic haemolytic anaemias
         — Pregnancy
         — Drugs (anticonvulsants, trimethoprim, methotrexate)
      (iii) Others (rare)
         — Lesch-Nyhan syndrome
         — Orotic aciduria
   (b) Normoblastic marrow
      — Alcohol (direct toxic effect)
      — Myxoedema
      — Hypopituitarism
      — Liver disease
      — Leukaemias, aplastic anaemia, myelosclerosis, sideroblastic anaemia
      — Bony metastases
      — Haemolysis, haemorrhage
      — Protein malnutrition
      — Scurvy
      — Down's syndrome
      — Drugs (azathioprine, cyclophosphamide)

Macrocytes are red cells with increased mean corpuscular volume, usually greater than 100 fl. Normal erythrocytes are about 7 μm in diameter. Macrocytes are 8–9 μm in diameter and may appear slightly oval-shaped in the peripheral blood film. Two-thirds of megaloblastic anaemias in the western world are due to auto-immune vitamin B_{12} deficiency. The presence of a hypersegmental neutrophil in this blood film suggests a megaloblastic cause.

Question 73

This is the skull radiograph of a 64-year-old patient.
What is the diagnosis?

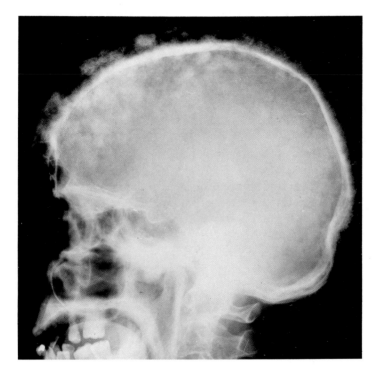

Answer to question 73

Paget's disease of the skull.

The highest incidence of Paget's disease is in Western Europe (particularly North England), occurring in 4% of the population over 50 years. It is often a chance radiological finding for most patients are asymptomatic.

This skull radiograph shows thickening of the calvarium with mixed lytic and sclerotic ('cotton-wool') areas. Rarely the lytic form of Paget's disease predominates in the calvarium, giving the sharply demarcated translucent osteoporosis circumscripta.

Paget's disease may affect any bone and in monostotic cases (single bone involvement), diagnostic difficulties may arise. The increased bone size and coarse trabeculae of Paget's disease help to distinguish this condition from an osteosclerotic metastasis. Furthermore, a bone survey may reveal other more typical areas of Paget's disease.

Question 74

This patient presented with fever, painful ankles and abdominal colic.
1. What is the diagnosis?
2. What is the treatment?

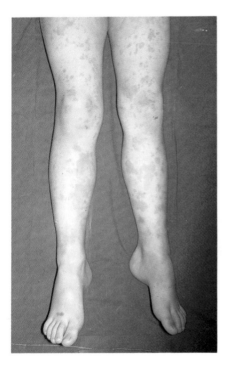

Answer to question 74

1. Henoch-Schönlein purpura.
2. Supportive only (corticosteroids for extensive bowel or joint involvement).

Henoch-Schönlein purpura is a condition of uncertain aetiology affecting principally the skin, joints, kidney and gastrointestinal tract. It is most frequently encountered in male children and most cases give a preceding history of upper respiratory tract infection. No micro-organism has been consistently associated with the condition and some attacks seem to be precipitated by allergy to drugs, food, insect stings, etc. The pathology is due to a disseminated arteriolar and capillary vasculitis, which is usually self-limiting.

The skin lesions are concentrated over the lower limbs and buttocks and are initially urticarial and macular (illustrated); non-thrombocytopenic purpura follows. The arthritis is temporary and tends to affect larger joints.

Abdominal pain from bowel haemorrhage and oedema may be severe, and in some cases intussusception occurs. About half of the cases have a focal proliferative nephritis with glomerular IgA and C_3 deposition. Serum IgA is raised but complement levels are normal.

For most patients the condition resolves completely, but a minority suffer a relapsing course and ultimately chronic renal failure. Corticosteroids are beneficial only for the joint and bowel manifestations.

Question 75

This patient presented with severe abdominal pain.
1. What two radiological abnormalities give the diagnosis in this tomogram?
2. What has happened?

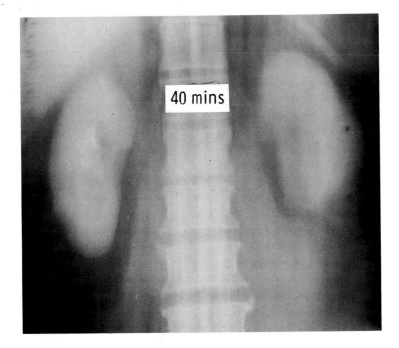

Answer to question 75

1. (a) Bilateral persistent dense nephrograms.
(b) Abdominal aortic aneurysm.
2. Dissecting aortic aneurysm causing reduced renal perfusion.

Immediate dense bilateral nephrograms which persist are usually due to acute tubular necrosis. Delayed bilateral nephrograms which become increasingly dense are seen in acute obstruction and renal ischaemia. In this case the renal artery orifices were compromised by the aneurysm and the IVU series showed increasingly dense nephrograms.

Question 76

1. What is this condition?
2. Give three other abnormalities that may be visible on inspection of the patient.

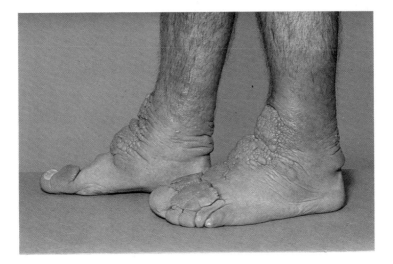

Answer to question 76

1. Pretibial myxoedema.
2. (a) Exophthalmos.
   (b) Goitre.
   (c) Acropachy.

Graves' disease occurs as a result of thyroid stimulating immunoglobulin adherence to the TSH receptor. This auto-immune condition is distinct from other causes of thyrotoxicosis (multinodular goitre, solitary nodule and thyroiditis) and is characterised by changes in other end-organs affected by the immune process.

Thyroid enlargement occurs in 10% of cases and is believed to be caused by a separate growth immunoglobulin. Skin and eye changes have similar aetiologies. Pretibial myxoedema can appear as diffuse non-pitting oedema over the shins or with circumscribed nodular and tuberous lesions.

Question 77

This is the blood film of a 5-year-old girl who presented with a maculopapular rash over the face and occipital lymphadenopathy.
1. What is the abnormal cell?
2. What is the diagnosis?

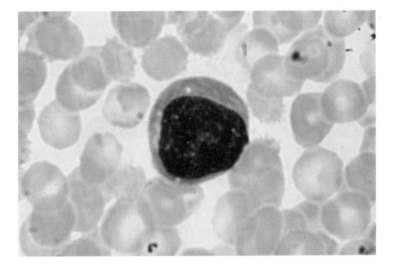

Answer to question 77

1. Turk cell (plasma cell with basophilic cytoplasm).
2. Rubella.

Rubella is caused by a spheroidal RNA virus. The typical presentation is with a maculopapular rash initially involving the forehead and face, and appearing 14–21 days after explosue to infection. In some cases outbreak of the rash is preceded by an influenza-like illness. Lymphadenopathy is usual, the posterior auricular and occipital nodes being the most commonly involved. Arthralgia and joint swelling occur more frequently in females than in males. Purpura and encephalomyelitis are rarer complications.

The characteristic haematological finding is a neutropenia with plasma cells in the peripheral circulation. Those with basophilic cytoplasm are known as Turk cells, and although common, they are not specific for this condition. In some cases there can be difficulty in differentiating these cells from the mononuclear cells of glandular fever. The diagnosis is made from the typical rash initially involving the face and can be confirmed by serological tests.

Routine vaccination of schoolgirls is available in order to reduce the incidence of congenital rubella. The vaccine should never be given in pregnancy.

Question 78

This is the CT scan of a 72-year-old alcoholic man who has become confused over the last five months.
What is the diagnosis?

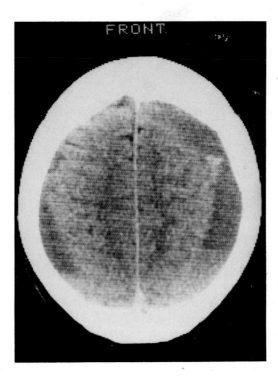

Answer to question 78

Chronic bilateral subdural haematomas.

The density of subdural collections on a CT scan give an indication of their age. In the acute stage the haematoma is of high density; it remains of higher attenuation than brain tissue for two weeks. Over the next four weeks the subdural collection becomes less dense than brain (as seen in this case). Because of this transition there is a period between two and four weeks when the subdural becomes isodense and it may be missed by the unwary. At this stage intravenous contrast may delineate the capsule of the haematoma, but this is not invariable.

Less than half of all patients with subdurals remember previous head injury and surprisingly trivial trauma may be responsible. Alcoholics are especially prone to subdurals, probably because of their liability to falls and impaired blood clotting.

The patient often presents with insidious mental changes which suggest either dementia or a primary intracranial lesion such as a frontal lobe tumour. Focal neurological signs and epilepsy are uncommon. A characteristic feature is fluctuation of the consciousness level, which may vary during the day from normal lucidity to extreme drowsiness.

Question 79

This girl returned from a Mediterranean holiday three weeks ago and now has developed these pruritic lesions.
1. What is the diagnosis?
2. What treatment is available?

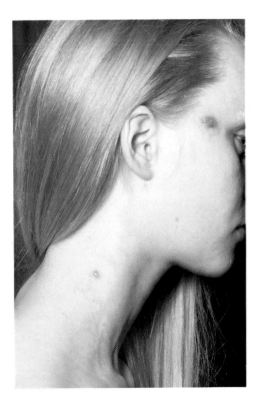

Answer to question 79

1. Cutaneous leishmaniasis.
2. Pentavalent antimonials.

'Old world' leishmaniasis is caused by *L. tropica*, a parasite of rodents and canines. The infection is spread by the sandfly (*Phlebotomus*) and is common in Africa, India and the Middle East, but may also be acquired in Mediterranean countries.

After an incubation period varying from a few days to six months a small pruritic papule develops at the site of inoculation. After scaling and crusting, a horny spicule may be found in the centre (Montpellier sign). Beneath the crust lies a shallow ulcer which slowly heals to leave a scar. The diagnosis may be confirmed with a biopsy revealing the characteristic appearance of intracellular Leishman-Donovan bodies.

The infection is limited by cell-mediated immunity, with the 'leishmanin' test becoming positive about three months after the appearance of the lesion. Serum antibodies remain undetectable throughout the illness.

Kala-azar (visceral leishmaniasis) is a different condition caused by *L. donovani*. Previous infection with *L. tropica* confers no resistance to it and the geographical distribution of the two diseases is distinct. Pentavalent antimonials are available for the treatment of kala-azar and the more disfiguring lesions of cutaneous leishmaniasis.

Question 80

These are the hands of a 26-year-old patient.
1. What are the two likely diagnoses?
2. Which single biochemical investigation will distinguish between them?

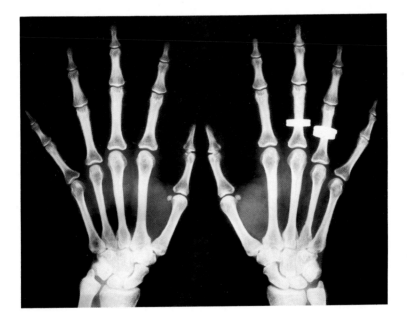

Answer to question 80

1. (a) Marfan's syndrome.
   (b) Homocystinuria.
2. Cyanide-nitroprusside test for urinary homocystine.

In both of these conditions there is elongation of the tubular bones, especially of the feet and hands. Both Marfan's syndrome and homocystinuria affect the cardiovascular and skeletal systems and cause ectopia lentis.

Marfan's syndrome is inherited as an autosomal dominant trait and has variable penetrance; the biochemical defect is unknown. The features of Marfan's syndrome are:

Eyes
— Upward lens dislocation (ectopia lentis); may result in glaucoma.
— Meiosis unresponsive to mydriatics.

Cardiovascular system
— Progressive dilatation of ascending aorta causes aortic incompetence and dissecting aneurysms.
— Atrial septal defects.
— Mitral valve prolapse.

Musculoskeletal system
— Tall, severe kyphoscoliosis.
— Pectus carinatum or excavatum.
— Arachnodactyly.
— High arched palate.
— Muscle hypotonia.
— Increased incidence of inguinal and femoral hernias.

Other features
— Sparse subcutaneous fat.
— Spontaneous pneumothorax.

Homocystinuria, which has recessive inheritance, shares most ocular and skeletal manifestations. Some differences found in homocystinuria are:
(i) Downward lens dislocation.
(ii) Mental retardation.
(iii) Arachnodactyly is less marked.
(iv) Osteoporosis.
(v) Vascular thrombosis is a frequent complication.

Question 81

1. What is this condition?
2. How is it inherited?
3. Give three complications.

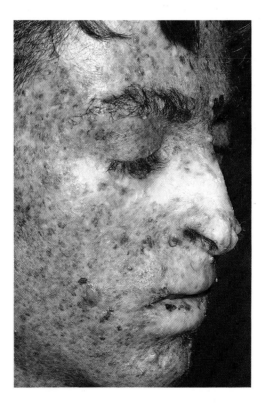

Answer to question 81

1. Xeroderma pigmentosum.
2. Autosomal recessive.
3. (a) Cutaneous malignancy.
   (b) Bone marrow failure.
   (c) Mental subnormality.

Xeroderma pigmentosum is an inherited disorder of DNA repair resulting in a cutaneous hypersensitivity to ultraviolet radiation. Premature ageing of the skin occurs, with freckling and atrophy. There is a greatly increased incidence of squamous and basal cell carcinoma and malignant melanoma. Most patients die in early adulthood from metastatic disease. Bone marrow and neurological disorders are common. The mainstay of therapy is protection from bright light and the use of high potency sun screens.

Question 82

What are the two radiological abnormalities?

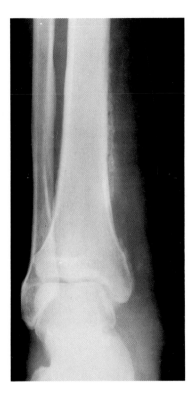

Answer to question 82

1. Loss of soft tissue due to ulceration.
2. Periosteal reaction.

Trauma, inflammation and primary neoplasms of bone are the commonest causes of a localised periosteal reaction. The clue to the cause of the granular periosteal reaction in this case is the irregular loss of soft tissue due to varicose ulceration.

The differential diagnosis of a periosteal reaction depends on whether it is localised or generalised. Causes of a localised periosteal reaction include:

(a) Trauma
(b) Infection
  — osteomyelitis
  — cellulitis
(c) Neoplastic
  — Benign, e.g. osteoid osteoma
  — Primary malignant, e.g. osteosarcoma, Ewing's sarcoma
  — Metastatic deposits (rare), e.g. neuroblastoma
(d) Polyarteritis nodosa
(e) Histiocytosis X.

Question 83

1. What is the diagnosis?
2. What three features typify this condition?
3. Name four signs that may be found on examination.

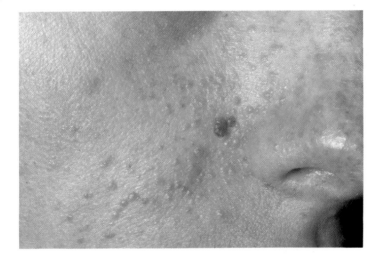

Answer to question 83

1. Tuberous sclerosis (epiloia).
2. (a) Adenoma sebaceum (illustrated).
   (b) Mental subnormality.
   (c) Convulsive seizures.
3. Physical signs include
   (a) Skin: shagreen patches (roughened patches of discoloured skin over the lower back); ash leaf patches (foliate regions of hypopigmentation); subungal fibromas.
   (b) Skeletal: spina bifida, syndactyly.
   (c) Eyes: cataract, retinal tumours and optic atrophy.

Tuberous sclerosis has an autosomal dominant mode of inheritance; the most serious pathology is found within the central nervous system. Regions of cortical malformation, consisting of monster nerve cells and glioblasts lie within the brain. These 'tubers' may calcify and be visible on plain skull radiographs.

Question 84

This patient was treated for a urinary tract infection and now has watery diarrhoea.
1. What does this biopsy of the sigmoid colon show?
2. How would you confirm the diagnosis?
3. How would you treat this patient?

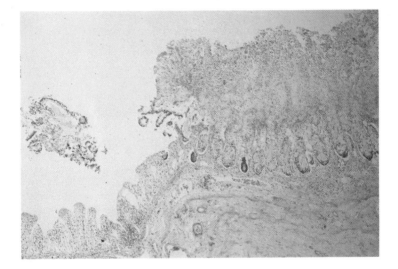

Answer to question 84

1. Pseudomembranous colitis (PMC).
2. Stool culture for *Clostridium difficile* and isolation of *Cl. difficile* toxin.
3. (a) Fluid and electrolyte replacement.
   (b) Oral vancomycin or metronidazole.

This biopsy shows a thick fibrinous membrane containing inflammatory cells. Under this 'pseudomembrane' the glands are distended and have lost their epithelial lining.

The features of PMC are abdominal pain and watery diarrhoea (very rarely the stools are bloody); these symptoms occur a few days after taking broad spectrum antibiotics. The typical pseudomembrane is not always seen on sigmoidoscopy and for this reason stools from patients with unexplained diarrhoea should be screened for *Cl. difficile* toxin to exclude PMC.

Treatment with oral vancomycin is usually rapidly effective. However, it is relatively expensive and unpalatable and a recent study has shown metronidazole to be equally effective.

Question 85

This patient complains of intermittent abdominal pain and bouts of diarrhoea.
1. What is the likely diagnosis?
2. How can this be confirmed?

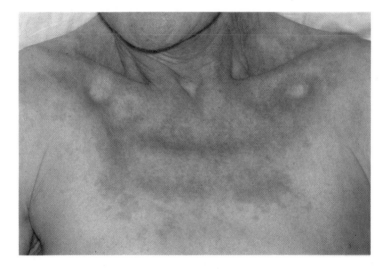

Answer to question 85

1. Carcinoid syndrome.
2. Elevated 24-hour urinary excretion of 5-hydroxyindoleacetic acid.

Carcinoid tumours arise from argentaffin cells and may secrete a variety of neurotransmitters and hormones, including 5HT (5-hydroxytryptamine), histamine, prostaglandins and vasoactive peptides. Attacks of flushing, abdominal pain and diarrhoea occur on systemic release of these agents. The flush is particularly prominent on the face and neck and other light exposed areas. Wheezing, tachycardia and hypotension may accompany an attack.

The primary tumour is usually found within the terminal ileum, but the gastric mucosa, biliary system, pancreas and lung are other recognised sites. With the exception of the rare ovarian primary, the syndrome does not occur without extensive metastatic spread.

Peritoneal, retroperitoneal and pleural fibrosis are additional complications and are found without evidence of local tumour. The endocardium may be similarly involved, leading to predominantly right-sided valvular lesions. Left-sided heart disease is a feature of bronchial carcinoids and in these cases the accompanying flush is said to be more severe and prolonged.

The tumours are slow-growing and treatment has traditionally been surgical, but there are reports of successful symptomatic control by the embolisation of hepatic secondary deposits. 5HT blockers, chlorpromazine and prostaglandin synthesis inhibitors can also reduce the severity of attacks. 5-hydroxyindoleacetic acid (a metabolite of 5HT) appears in the urine in excess and provides a useful diagnostic test for the disease and a marker for response to tumour-ablative treatment.

Question 86

1. What does this barium study show?
2. How would you treat this patient?

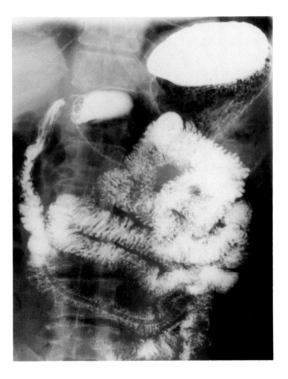

Answer to question 86

1. *Ascaris lumbricoides* in the jejunum.
2. Oral piperazine, levamisole or pyrantel.

Ascariasis is found worldwide but is commonest in Africa and the Far East. There are two stages of the infection, and the stage determines the clinical features. Larval ascariasis is the first phase and is caused by the migration of ingested larvae from the intestine to the lungs via the liver; the resulting respiratory symptoms are cough, wheezing and sometimes haemoptysis. The larvae then pass up the bronchioles to the trachea and spill over into the pharynx. The larvae then mature in the gut; this is the adult worm phase. The severity of the clinical manifestations at this stage depends on how heavy the infestation is: a light infection is asymptomatic. Mild infection causes abdominal colic. Heavier worm loads may result in volvulus, obstruction and perforation. In the tropics, children with heavy infections are malnourished and a plain abdominal radiograph may show the 'Medusa's lock' sign of gas trapped between a mass of worms. Further migration of the worms within the gut may cause pancreatitis, cholecystitis and appendicitis. The diagnosis usually relies on the finding of *Ascaris* eggs in the patient's stools.

The most widely used treatment is oral piperazine. This drug paralyses the worms, which are then passed in the stool. Most of the drugs currently used for ascariasis can be given as a single dose.

Question 87

This patient has had a splenectomy.
1. What abnormality is present?
2. Name one other cause of this appearance.

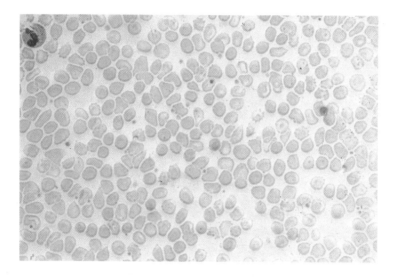

Answer to question 87

1. Howell-Jolly bodies.
2. (a) Splenic atrophy
  — Coeliac disease
  — Sickle cell anaemia.
  (b) Dyshaemopoietic states
  — Megaloblastic anaemia
  — Leukaemia

Howell-Jolly bodies are identified in erythrocytes as eccentrically placed fragments of nuclear material, about 1 μm in diameter. Although a common finding in the erythroid cells of the bone marrow, they are rarely seen in the peripheral blood.

They are pitted from erythrocytes in the splenic sinusoids, as are Heinz and Bartonella bodies. Following splenectomy there is an acute rise in the leucocyte and platelet count, and target and nucleated red cells may be found in the peripheral circulation. Within a few weeks these changes disappear leaving only an excess of erythrocyte Howell-Jolly bodies. The indications for splenectomy include trauma, hereditary spherocytosis, idiopathic thrombocytopenic purpura and occasionally for myelosclerosis, chronic leukaemias and acquired haemolytic anaemias.

Children with splenic atrophy or following splenectomy are particularly at risk of infection from encapsulated bacteria. Pneumococcal vaccine is recommended for these patients.

Question 88

1. What is this condition?
2. Name three causes.

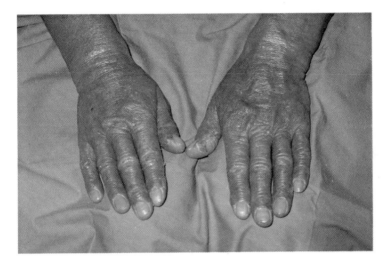

Answer to question 88

1. Erythroderma (exfoliative dermatitis).
2. (a) Eczema.
   (b) Psoriasis.
   (c) Leukaemia and reticuloses.
   (d) Drugs (gold, penicillin, barbiturates).

Erythroderma is an exfoliative dermatitis of universal distribution; typically the exfoliation is clinically inconspicuous. The condition is twice as common in men as in women and the majority of patients are over the age of 45. Histologically the dermis is oedematous and infiltrated with inflammatory cells.

Most cases are secondary to eczema or psoriasis, particularly following the use of systemic steroids. The Sézary syndrome, a T-cell 'leukaemic' variant of mycosis fungoides, presents with erythroderma.

Question 89

This patient presented with painful hips.
1. What is the diagnosis?
2. Name four predisposing causes.

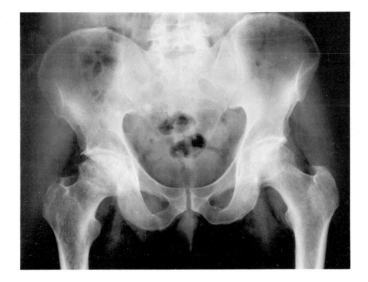

Answer to question 89

1. Avascular necrosis of the femoral heads.
2. (a) Iatrogenic: irradiation, steroid therapy.
  (b) Haematological disorders: sickle-cell disease, polycythaemia, macroglobulinaemia, haemophilia.
  (c) Connective tissue diseases: rheumatoid arthritis, SLE.
  (d) High pressure environments: caisson disease.
  (e) Trauma: subcapital fracture.
  Rarer causes include Gaucher's disease, pancreatitis, chronic alcoholism and pregnancy.

When the arterial supply of a bone-end is occluded, for whatever reason, there is a considerable delay (up to two years) before any radiological change is visible. The radiological features of established avascular necrosis are sclerosis of the subchondral bone with irregularity of the articular surface and, rarely, fragmentation of the bone.

Question 90

1. What is this lesion?
2. Name two complications.

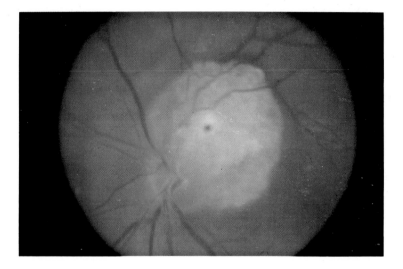

Answer to question 90

1. Drüsen of the optic nerve head.
2. (a) Visual field defects.
   (b) Retinal haemorrhage.

Drüsen are hyaline deposits found beneath the retinal pigment layer or in the optic nerve head. They are often bilateral, and have an incidence of about 3 per 1000. The inheritance is dominant. Disc lesions have an irregular scalloped edge giving the typical 'grape cluster' appearance. The condition is usually benign but disruption of nerve fibres may lead to visual field defects. The macula is seldom involved. An increase in large vessels at the disc with abnormal branching patterns predisposes to retinal haemorrhage.

In some cases fluorescein angiography may be required to distinguish this condition from papilloedema. Drüsen remain unstained, but with papilloedema there is persistent fluorescence.

Question 91

1. What is the diagnosis?
2. Name four haematological abnormalities which may be associated with this condition?

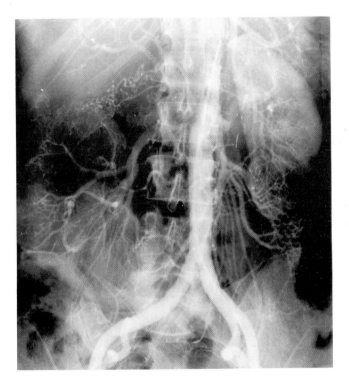

Answer to question 91

1. Hypernephroma of the right kidney.
2. (a) Anaemia in 50% (usually normocytic normochromic).
   (b) Erythrocytosis in 5%.
   (c) Eosinophilia.
   (d) Thrombocytosis.
   (e) Leukaemoid reaction.
   (f) Plasmacytosis.
   (g) Raised ESR.

This arteriogram shows a mass occupying the upper pole of the right kidney. Pathological vessels are seen entering its superior aspect. A simple renal cyst would appear avascular with normal vessels stretched over its surface. Arteriography has largely been abandoned in favour of ultrasound and CT scans in the investigation of a renal mass.

Hypernephromas account for 2% of all adult neoplasms. The triad of loin pain, abdominal mass and haematuria is in fact an uncommon presentation of a hypernephroma. In addition to the haematological abnormalities there are many other ways in which a hypernephroma may present:

(a) Fever.
(b) Weight loss, malaise.
(c) Hypercalcaemia (bone metastases or PTH production).
(d) Nephrotic syndrome.
(e) Secondary amyloidosis.
(f) Varicocele, IVC thrombosis or Budd-Chiari syndrome due to venous thrombosis.
(g) Ectopic hormone production (e.g. prolactin, renin, glucocorticoids, gonadotrophins).
(h) Symptomatic metastases, usually bone and lung.

Question 92

This patient presented with an influenza-like illness and now has become confused with a disproportionate bradycardia.
1. What is the likely diagnosis?
2. Name two tests that will confirm this.
3. What treatment is necessary?

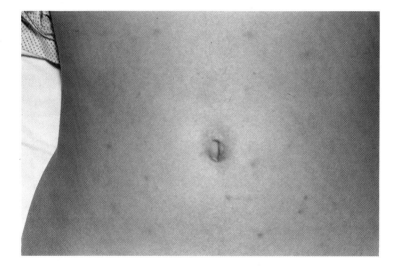

Answer to question 92

1. Typhoid (enteric) fever.
2. (a) Direct isolation of organism:
     — Blood culture (80–90% positive, even higher yield from marrow).
     — Stool culture (80% positive).
     — Culture from rose spot (60% positive).
     — Urine culture (25% positive).
   (b) Serology:
     — *Salmonella* agglutinins (Widal test) – only 50% positive at this stage.
3. Chloramphenicol; co-trimoxazole and ampicillin for milder cases.

The severity of human salmonellosis may vary from an asymptomatic carrier state to life-threatening typhoid fever; most patients suffer from a gastroenteritis.

Typhoid fever is caused by *Salmonella typhi* and strains of *paratyphi*. These organisms are highly adapted to man and have no other reservoir in nature. The clinical course of the disease may be considered in four stages.

During the incubation period (1–2 weeks) patients have an influenza-like illness, occasionally with a gastroenteritis. The second stage is characterised by constipation, hepatosplenomegaly, lymphadenopathy and encephalopathy. Ileal perforation can occur and rose spots (illustrated) are seen over the abdominal wall. A relative bradycardia is typical.

Metastatic infection, immune complex nephritis and myocarditis are features of the third stage. Finally a carrier state is defined for those patients still harbouring the organism one year after the initial illness. The biliary tree is the usual site, particularly if there are underlying structural abnormalities.

The diagnosis is made from blood and stool culture and serology. However, the Widal test is only positive in about 50% of cases during the acute phase of the illness and false positives may occur with chronic active hepatitis and connective tissue diseases. During convalescence up to 80% become positive.

Question 93

This is the bone marrow biopsy of a 34-year-old patient with lymphadenopathy.
1. What does the biopsy show?
2. What is the likely diagnosis?
3. Name four haematological abnormalities you might find in this condition.

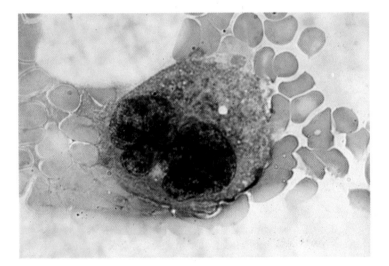

Answer to question 93

1. Reed-Sternberg cell.
2. Hodgkin's disease.
3. (a) Normochromic normocytic anaemia.
   (b) Autoimmune haemolytic anaemia.
   (c) Leucoerythroblastic anaemia.
   (d) Neutrophil leucocytosis.
   (e) Eosinophilia.
   (f) Monocytosis.
   (g) Lymphopenia.
   (h) Raised platelet count, reduced in later stages.
   (i) Raised ESR.

The diagnosis of Hodgkin's disease cannot be made without the finding of Reed-Sternberg cells in either a lymph node or bone marrow biopsy. In addition, to fulfil the histological criteria for Hodgkin's disease, there must be neoplastic reticulum cells and destruction of lymph node architecture. The Reed-Sternberg cell is large, irregular and has a complicated bi-lobed nucleus with prominent nucleoli. The abundance of these cells varies with the histological type of Hodgkin's lymphoma.

The haematological state of the patient depends largely on the extent of bone marrow infiltration. The activity of the disease correlates well with the neutrophil alkaline phosphatase score and the ESR.

Question 94

From what multisystem disease is this patient suffering?

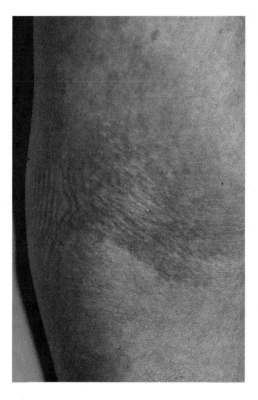

Answer to question 94

Pseudoxanthoma elasticum.

This is an inherited disorder of elastic tissue usually transmitted as an autosomal recessive trait. Females are affected more severely than males. Yellow, papular lesions (pseudoxanthomas) may develop on the skin of the neck, axillae, antecubital fossae and groins; they are usually apparent by the second decade.

Other systems involved include:

Eyes. A deficiency in the elastic tissue of Bruch's membrane gives the fundoscopic appearance of angioid streaks. These are flat and dark red in colour. They lie beneath the retinal vessels and appear to emanate from the disc (a similar appearance may be found with Paget's disease, sickle cell anaemia and the Ehlers-Danlos syndrome). Neovascularisation and haemorrhage can cause significant visual loss.

Gastrointestinal tract. Upper gastrointestinal haemorrhage may be the presenting feature, and in these cases it may be difficult to identify the source of blood loss.

Cardiovascular system. Premature arterial degeneration and calcification causes claudication, angina pectoris and hypertension.

Question 95

1. What is the diagnosis?
2. Name two other clinical features of this condition.

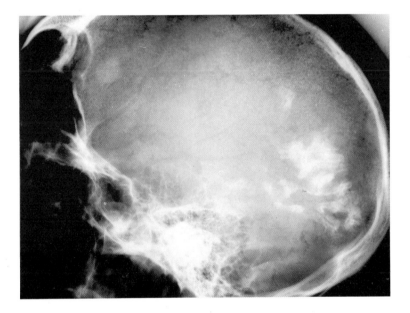

Answer to question 95

1. Sturge-Weber syndrome.
2. (a) Port wine stain in a sensory branch distribution of the trigeminal nerve.
   (b) Focal epilepsy.
   (c) Visual field defect (due to occipital lobe lesion).

The Sturge-Weber syndrome consists of a capillary haemangioma within the cutaneous distribution of the trigeminal nerve and a venous haemangioma of the meninges. These lesions are ipsilateral and the first neurological manifestation is usually a focal epileptic fit on the opposite side to the skin naevus.

The intracranial calcification showing a convoluted 'rail road' appearance is diagnostic of Sturge-Weber syndrome. This pattern is due to calcification of sulci overlying atrophic brain rather than calcification of the angiomatous vessels.

The diagnosis is usually obvious and angiography is rarely necessary. These patients have a normal life expectancy although they may have permanent neurological deficits and mental retardation. Treatment is aimed at controlling the often intractable epilepsy with anticonvulsants. The lesions are usually too extensive to allow surgical removal.

Question 96

1. What is this condition?
2. What is the commonest cause?

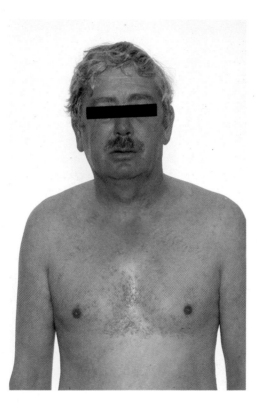

Answer to question 96

1. Superior vena cava obstruction (superior mediastinal syndrome).
2. Occlusion of the superior vena cava from mediastinal extension of a carcinoma at the right hilum.

The clinical features are those of venous engorgement of the upper body, facial congestion and oedema. There is static elevation of the jugular venous pressure and prominence of fine veins around the chest wall and at the costal margins. There may be a history of headache, or occasionally vertigo.

Rarer causes of SVC obstruction include (a) lymphoma (b) retrosternal thyroid (c) aortic aneurysm (d) idiopathic fibrosing mediastinitis (associated with retroperitoneal fibrosis; some cases have been reported after methysergide therapy).

Question 97

1. What is the likely diagnosis?
2. Name four conditions affecting the liver that are associated with this disease.

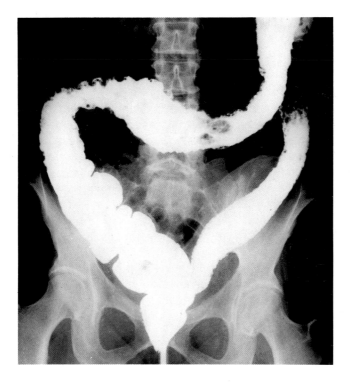

Answer to question 97

1. Ulcerative colitis.
2. (a) Fatty change.
   (b) Chronic active hepatitis.
   (c) Cirrhosis.
   (d) Amyloidosis.
   (e) Pericholangitis.
   (f) Sclerosing cholangitis.
   (g) Bile duct carcinoma.

There are two features of this single contrast 'instant' enema which help to make the distinction between ulcerative colitis and Crohn's disease. In this case the fine mucosal ulceration (transmural and 'rose thorn' in Crohn's disease) extends continuously from the rectum to the transverse colon; Crohn's disease is often discontinuous, giving rise to skip lesions. Rectal involvement, seen here, is an almost invariable finding in ulcerative colitis. In Crohn's disease the proximal colon is more commonly affected and the rectum is frequently spared.

The liver diseases found in association with ulcerative colitis and Crohn's disease are similar but sclerosing cholangitis is very rarely seen in Crohn's disease and the incidence of gall-stones is only increased in Crohn's disease.

Question 98

This is the echocardiogram of a patient who presented with shortness of breath.
1. What abnormality can be seen?
2. What is the cause?

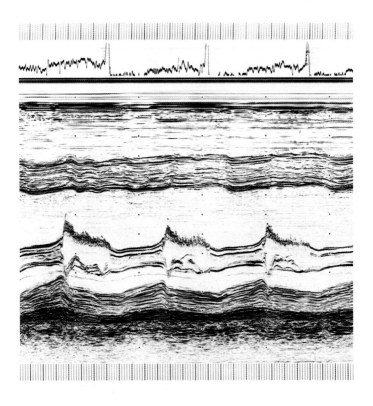

Answer to question 98

1. Flutter on anterior leaflet of mitral valve.
2. Aortic regurgitation.

The cardinal echocardiographic sign of aortic regurgitation is the appearance of a high frequency flutter superimposed on the anterior leaflet echo of the mitral valve during diastole. This is believed to be a consequence of the cusp's position in relation to the regurgitant stream of blood beneath the aortic root. Such a mechanism does not explain fully the apical diastolic rumble often heard in this condition.

Austin Flint believed this murmur to be caused by a relative mitral stenosis as the valve leaflets drifted together early in diastole because of a rapid pressure rise from double ventricular filling. In long-standing aortic regurgitation with left ventricular cavity dilatation this pressure rise does not occur. However, the mechanism accounts for the echocardiographic finding of premature mitral valve closure in acute aortic insufficiency and the clinical detection of a soft first heart sound in both this condition and acute mitral regurgitation.

Another theory has suggested that the Austin Flint murmur is merely an apical transmission of the low frequency components of the murmur at the aortic valve, as in some cases the rumble arises immediately after the second sound, before mitral valve opening can occur. The most generally accepted explanation is that the regurgitant aortic flow becomes deviated onto the under surface of the mitral valve, resulting in a relative mitral stenosis.

Question 99

1. What is the likely underlying disorder?
2. Name four causes.

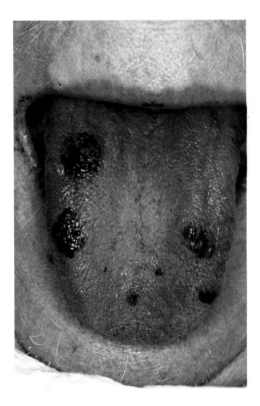

Answer to question 99

1. Thrombocytopenia.
2. (a) Myelosuppression (drugs, chemicals).
  (b) Autoimmune (idiopathic thrombocytopenic purpura, systemic lupus erythematosus, drugs).
  (c) Marrow aplasia and infiltrations.
  (d) Reduced platelet survival (disseminated intravascular coagulation).
  (e) Disorders of platelet function (hereditary, uraemia).

Haemorrhagic bullae on the tongue and mucous membranes are virtually pathognomonic of thrombocytopenia.
Frequently the disorder is iatrogenic. Cytotoxic agents, thiazides, oestrogens, penicillins, sulphonamides, oral hypoglycaemics and salicylates are some of the recognised causes.
  Acute idiopathic thrombocytopenic purpura is more common in children and is associated with the adherence of IgG and C_3 to the platelet membrane. Severe cases may require glucocorticoids and splenectomy, or paradoxically, cytotoxic therapy. Fresh platelet transfusions provide temporary benefit in the event of haemorrhage.

Question 100

This is the chest radiograph of a 68-year-old woman who presented with recurrent episodes of breathlessness.
1. Name three abnormalities.
2. What is the diagnosis?

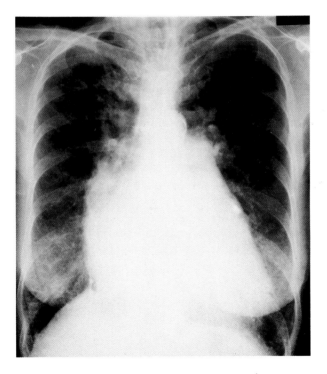

Answer to question 100

1. (a) Cardiomegaly.
   (b) Left atrial enlargement with calcified appendage.
   (c) Interstitial pulmonary oedema (Kerley B lines).
2. Rheumatic mitral valve disease.

Deciding which chamber is enlarged from a chest radiograph showing cardiomegaly is difficult and often unreliable.

There is a double right heart border in this radiograph, implying left atrial enlargement. Other radiological signs of left atrial enlargement are splaying of the carina and posterior displacement of a barium-filled oesophagus.

Left atrial size correlates well with the severity of mitral incompetence whereas in mitral stenosis the size of the left atrium bears little relation to the severity of the stenosis; the appearance of interstitial pulmonary oedema (which reflects left atrial pressure) is a more reliable sign of the degree of stenosis.

Long-standing raised left atrial pressure may result in mottling of the lung fields due to pulmonary haemosiderosis and rarely small foci of bone are seen in the mid and lower zones.

Question 101

1. What is this condition?
2. What is the underlying disease?
3. Give three other eye changes seen in this disease.

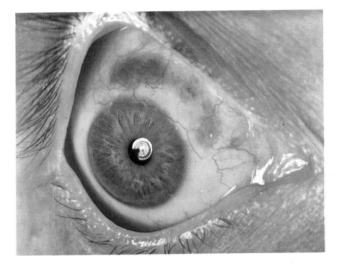

Answer to question 101

1. Scleromalacia.
2. Rheumatoid arthritis.
3. (a) Episcleritis.
    (b) Scleritis.
    (c) Keratitis.
    (d) Keratoconjunctivitis sicca.

Episcleritis appears as a mild injection at the limbus, and is usually asymptomatic. Scleritis is less common and causes an acutely painful red eye which may progress to ulceration. Subsequent scleral atrophy (scleromalacia) allows the blue colour of the underlying choroid to become visible. Glaucoma, cataract and retinal detachment are other complications. Long-standing rheumatoid arthritis sufferers, particularly women, may develop scleromalacia in the absence of a preceding scleritis. In these circumstances the lesions are frequently bilateral.

Atrophy of the lacrimal glands results in keratoconjunctivitis sicca. With salivary involvement, dryness of the mouth occurs (xerostomia). The triad of keratoconjunctivitis sicca, xerostomia and rheumatoid arthritis is known as 'Sjögren's syndrome'.

Iritis is an unusual feature of rheumatoid disease and is more typically associated with the seronegative arthropathies.

Index